Regie's Rainbow Adventure®

National Kidney Foundation of Michigan's nutrition education program for disease prevention in the early childcare setting

Copyright © 2016 by National Kidney Foundation of Michigan

All Rights Reserved. This material is based upon work supported by the Corporation for National and Community Service (CNCS) under Grant No. 11SIHMI001. Opinions or points of view expressed in this document are those of the authors and do not necessarily reflect the official position of, or a position that is endorsed by, CNCS or the CNCS's Social Innovation Fund. The Social Innovation Fund is a program of the CNCS, a federal agency that engages more than 5 million Americans in service through its AmeriCorps, Senior Corps, Social Innovation Fund, and Volunteer Generation Fund programs, and leads the President's national call to service initiative, United We Serve. Learn more at nationalservice.gov/Innovation.

This book was created in partnership with United Way for Southeastern Michigan (UWSEM), which facilitated the CNCS grant in the Detroit area. Opinions or points of view expressed in this book are those of the authors and do not necessarily reflect the official position of UWSEM. Copyrighted UWSEM logos and texts are used with the organization's permission. All rights reserved.

Regie's Rainbow Adventure® is a registered trademark of the National Kidney Foundation of Michigan. For more information, contact us at:
Author address: 1169 Oak Valley Drive, Ann Arbor, MI 48108
Web domain: www.nkfm.org

All rights reserved. This book or any portion thereof may not be reproduced or used in any manner without the express written permission of the National Kidney Foundation of Michigan. This book is intended as a reference. It is not intended to be used to duplicate any part of the Regie's Rainbow Adventure program which is copyrighted by the National Kidney Foundation of Michigan. Should you wish to bring the program, or part of it, to your community, please contact the National Kidney Foundation of Michigan for details on permission.
www.nkfm.org   800-482-1455

For more information and further discussion, visit

BibToBackpack.org

ISBN: 978-1-942011-64-4

Cover art and design by Rick Nease www.RickNeaseArt.com

Publishing services provided by Front Edge Publishing, LLC

For information about customized editions, bulk purchases or permissions, contact Front Edge Publishing, LLC at info@FrontEdgePublishing.com

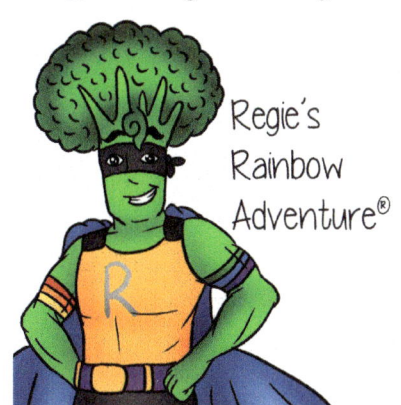

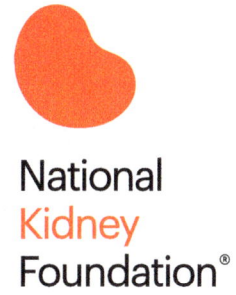

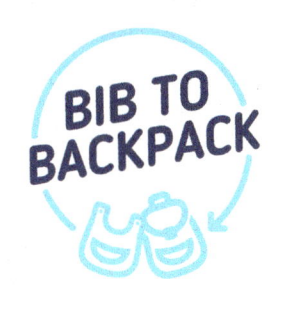

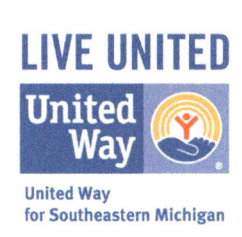

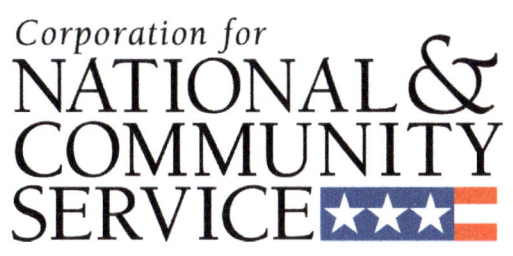

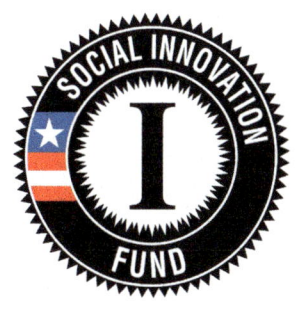

Contents

Preface ix
Introduction xiii

CHAPTER 1: WELCOME! 1

CHAPTER 2: OUR STORY 5
   Up! Up and Away! A Morning With Regie 6
   Confronting the Challenge in Childhood 16
   The Regie Bag 24
   Regie Comes to Life 26
   Going on Regie's Adventure 35
   Regie's Real Superpower 45
   It's a Bird! It's a Plane! It's Regie! 58

CHAPTER 3: OUR RESOURCES 61
   Want to Become Regie? 62
   Eating the colors of the rainbow 65
   Recommended Websites 65
   Warm Sweet Potato and Apple Bake 66
   Carrot Cake Oatmeal Cookies 67

CHAPTER 4: OUR PARTNERS 69
   Tips from United Way and the Social Innovation Fund . 71
   Why United Way is an effective partner 76
   Tips from our portfolio evaluator 79

CHAPTER 5: ACKNOWLEDGEMENTS 83
   About the Authors 85
   The Bib to Backpack Learning Series 86

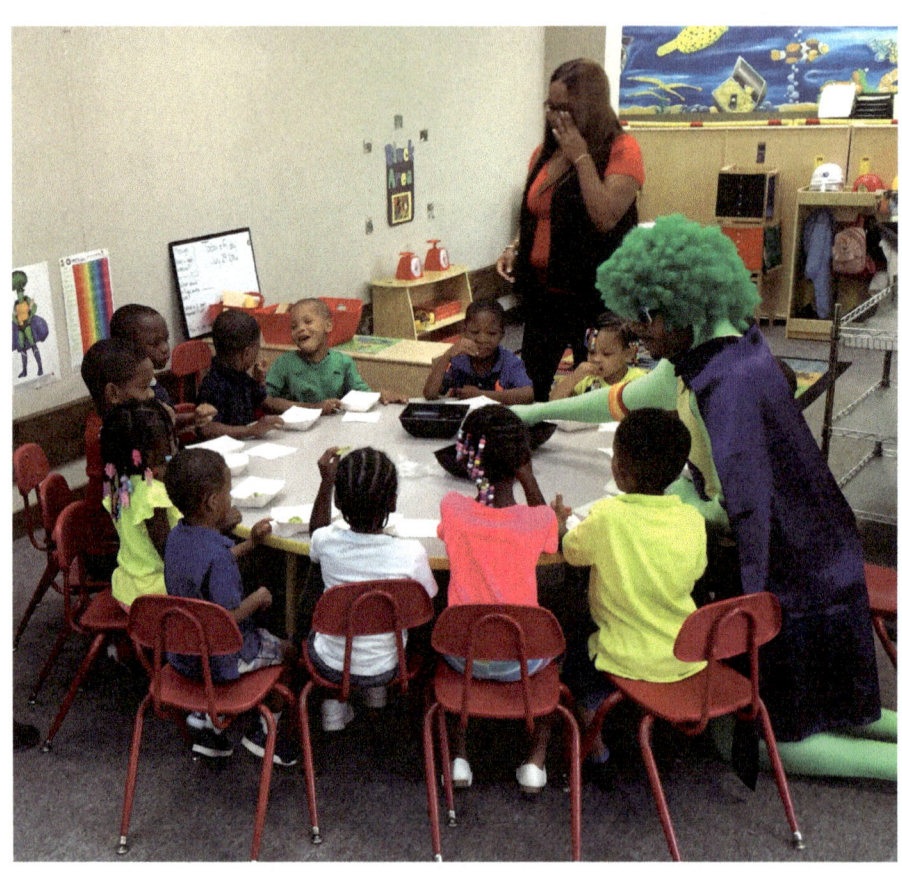

Regie visits young friends in a Detroit classroom and samples some green fruits and vegetables.

The National Kidney Foundation of Michigan would like to dedicate this book to the children and families who have taken this magical journey with Regie. They have traveled from the Island of Red all the way to the Island of Purple. With Regie's help, they've become healthier and have developed a new excitement for eating fruits and vegetables.

We also dedicate this book to all of our early childhood partners who implemented Regie's Rainbow Adventure® and transformed their classrooms into enchanted places of healthy eating and active movement.

This adventure of trying new healthy foods, gaining power stripes and singing our way through the rainbow would not have been possible without all of you! Through these adventures, we have learned that our bodies are healthiest when our plates are filled with an assortment of colorful fruits and vegetables. Our families and partners have truly been instrumental in ensuring that our children continue to fuel their bodies by eating healthy foods and by increasing physical activity. Thanks to your continued support and dedication, our children will live healthier lives.

"With every healthy meal and snack you provide for kids in your community, you're not just nourishing them today; you are shaping their habits and their tastes for the rest of their lives."

—Michelle Obama

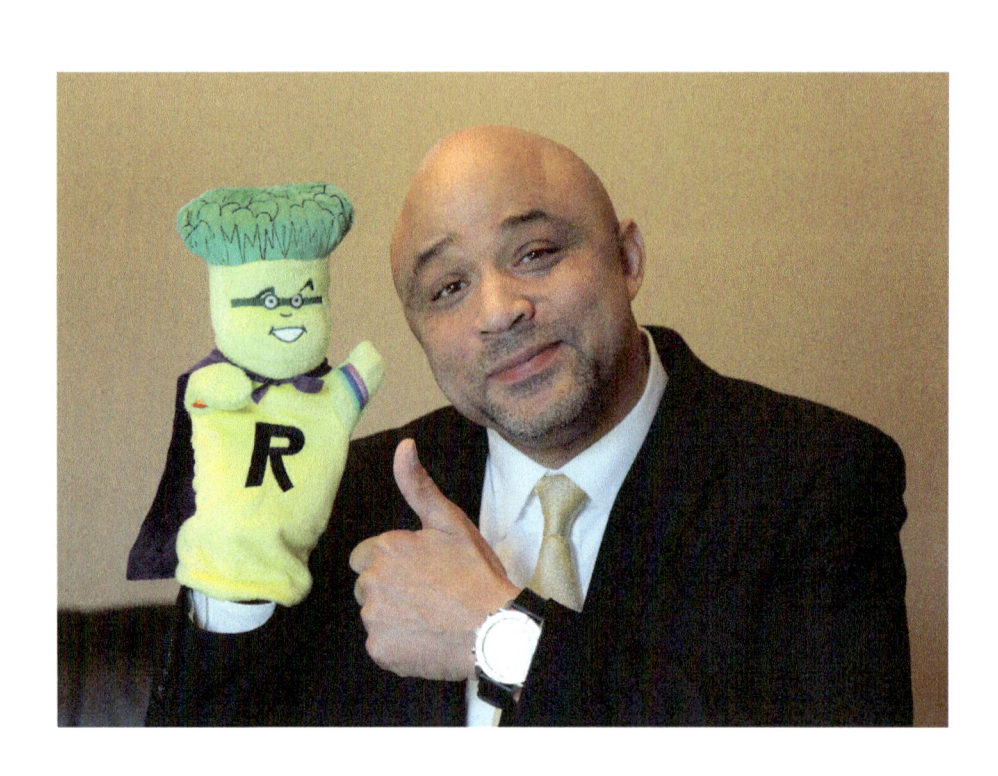

Preface

By Morris W. Hood III

Each child's life is the beginning of our future.

In our world today, we could find ourselves distracted by the many obstacles we face and we could forget about the health and education of our children. But, we cannot let that happen. Early childhood education and health go hand in hand in raising children to reach their full potential. We know that their success is truly our success as they become our next generation of leaders. If we give our children a strong and healthy head start now, they will help us build a better world.

I learned this lesson at a young age. When I was growing up, families all lent a helping hand. People knew they had to reach down and grab us up as children to help us forward. As adults today, we may not even remember all the adults who helped us along the way, but we must remember they were there. When we say it takes a village to raise a child, that's the kind of experience many of us had with relatives and neighbors as we were growing up. What the National Kidney Foundation of Michigan is doing with Regie's Rainbow Adventure® is a huge step in the right direction for children today. It's an experience all of us can give to our kids that they will remember throughout their lives. It's an early experience that ultimately will help them to achieve success in this challenging world we live in today.

I'm proud to be part of a family that has been concerned about the well-being and futures of children and their families for several generations. My grandfather, Morris Sr., and his brother, William, came to Detroit from Georgia and were involved in the early years of the labor movement, trying to protect the livelihood of working families. My father, Morris Jr., and his brother, Raymond Sr., were state legislators who always advocated for education and ways that we could equip our children for a great future. All my life, I've watched my family work toward these goals in ways that ranged from large to small. And that's something I appreciate about Regie's program: It covers a broad range of topics, and works directly with families to help them in their homes, promoting nutrition and physical activity. That's how we must work: one family at a time.

This is personal for me. When I was a child of 10, I was diagnosed with type 1 diabetes. Now, I've lived with diabetes for more than 40 years. Diabetes changed my world at a very early age as I became insulin dependent. Growing up as a child, there was a special diet that I had to follow. When I went to camp, a relative's house or a friend's house for sleepovers—we had to remember my dietary needs. Diabetes affects your whole life and Regie is an excellent role model to help people take care of themselves, their health, and to form a positive nutritional outlook.

So, I'm strongly committed to effective programs like Regie's Rainbow Adventure that foster a healthy lifestyle of eating good foods and making sure you get more physical activity. The National Kidney Foundation of Michigan is doing something very important with Regie and we need to continue to support this effort. When it comes to these health issues: Knowledge truly is power.

Let me put this in language kids can appreciate: *Regie is cool! Eating fruits and vegetables with Regie is cool!* We just enjoy thinking about how strong and healthy we're getting by following Regie's advice. Regie brings smiles to everyone's faces—children *and* adults.

The National Kidney Foundation of Michigan gave me a puppet of Regie and I know that you just have to smile when you see him come to life. In fact, I found myself experimenting with different voices for Regie when I was playing with my young nieces and nephews. That's why this program is so successful. It's so much fun for children, their families and adults too!

But, don't mistake healthy eating and wellness for a minor issue. We know that providing the best educational programs in the world to our children isn't going to be successful if our children aren't showing up for school healthy and ready to learn. So many studies are showing us what a lack of good nutrition, too many sugary foods and a lack of physical activity are doing to this generation of children. We all want to improve education in this country. We should start by ensuring that our children are healthy, active and ready to learn.

Regie is there through that entire process. First, he's teaching us about eating more fruits and vegetables. Then, he's showing us how important it is to be physically active. We've all seen the studies showing a dramatic increase in the amount of screen time for kids today. We've all seen kids sitting and watching TV and, when they're not in front of the TV, they are playing games on some other digital device. Once children get to know Regie, they will want to leap tall buildings in a single bound like our hero. They will want to get active and move around—running, playing and participating in all of the activities that lead to a happy life.

I see many signs of encouragement in the health of the communities we serve in Michigan. In Detroit, urban gardening and agribusinesses are taking off and providing innovative healthy food in ways that we have never seen before. I'm also very proud of Detroit's Eastern Market, one of the oldest and largest year-round markets in the United States, where fresh fruits and vegetables from farmers—from all over the world—come together in our community. There are many signs of hope—and Regie is one of those encouraging signs!

Remember this: Education and health go hand in hand to help build a successful future for all of us. Together, we can make a difference.

Senator Morris W. Hood III *was elected to three terms in the Michigan House of Representatives and was elected in both 2010 and 2014 to the Michigan Senate. Among his top legislative priorities are education and public health.*

Introduction

By Ken Resnicow, Ph.D.

The Regie's Rainbow Adventure® program addresses two vital public health issues amongst our youth: healthy eating and physical activity. Children living in lower-resource neighborhoods have disproportionately higher rates of obesity and other chronic diseases, including type 2 diabetes, hypertension, hyperlipidemia and sleep apnea. Moreover, overweight children are more than five times as likely as their healthy counterparts to have a lower health-related quality of life and impaired psychologic functioning. A poor early childhood health status also predicts lower academic achievement in subsequent schooling. Moreover, healthy children miss less school.

These risks can be greatly diminished with early intervention. Programs that encourage healthy eating and physical activity can reduce the risk of obesity and its many physical, psychological and social consequences.

As noted by the World Health Organization, "early childhood development is considered to be the most important phase in life which determines the quality of health, well-being, learning and behavior across the life span."

This viewpoint is further reflected in the U.S. Department of Health and Human Services Healthy People 2020 report, that states: "Evidence shows that experiences in early and middle childhood are extremely important for a child's healthy development and lifelong learning. How a child develops during this time affects future cognitive, social, emotional and physical development, which in turn influences school readiness and later success in life. Research on a number of adult health and medical conditions points to pre-disease pathways that have their beginnings in early and middle childhood."

It is important to note that Regie's Rainbow Adventure programming takes place in the childcare center, a setting that is ideal yet under-utilized for health interventions, when taking into consideration the large percentage of children served through childcare and the amount of time per day that many children spend there. Approximately 60 percent of preschool-aged children in the United States spend time in some type of childcare setting, spending an average of 29 hours per week in non-parental care (*The State of America's Children®, 2010*).

Providing programming to low-income childcare centers, like Head Start preschools, reaches particularly vulnerable populations who are most in need of health interventions. Regie's Rainbow Adventure encourages children to eat healthy and be more active in a fun and positive way—through the use of a superhero role model. Students, parents and teachers find this program engaging and worthwhile. Regie's Rainbow Adventure is helping to create a generation of healthy learners, with the ultimate potential of improving educational and health outcomes by setting children up for a healthier and more productive life.

Ken Resnicow, Ph.D, *is the Irwin M. Rosenstock collegiate professor of health behavior and health education at the University of Michigan School of Public Health and a professor of pediatrics in the School of Medicine.*

Welcome!

By Daniel Carney and Linda Smith-Wheelock

As the prevalence of obesity in children increases, so does the rate of type 2 diabetes, which is a leading cause of kidney failure. One in three children who were born in 2000 will develop diabetes in their lifetime. These startling statistics are what drove the National Kidney Foundation of Michigan (NKFM) to dedicate the last decade to providing nutrition education for low-income, preschool-aged children and their families. We know that teaching children healthy habits at an early age can prepare them for success later in life.

The National Kidney Foundation of Michigan offers a wide variety of innovative and creative early childhood health education programs. Our Project for EArly Childhood Health (PEACH) programs educate and empower families, childcare providers, teachers and children to make healthy changes in their schools, early childcare centers and homes. These programs reach those most in need—children and families from schools and neighborhoods that lack healthy food access, sound nutritional information and other vital health-related resources.

Regie's Rainbow Adventure® is one of our PEACH programs and is a direct answer to the childhood obesity problem. This program educates preschool children on the benefits of healthy eating and physical activity, with the goal of increasing fruit and vegetable consumption and creating positive attitudes about healthy behaviors. By implementing the Regie program, teachers are empowered to become role models through a fun, easy-to-use curriculum that creates a healthy classroom. This type of positive, active learning—made simple through the classroom-based curriculum—is behavior-changing in the low-income, vulnerable communities where it is implemented. We also measure outcomes through this program, including changes in physical-activity-related behaviors; amounts of screen time; consumption of sugar-sweetened beverages and fruits and vegetables in general; and general health indicators. All of these goals are set and met through a fun superhero named Regie, who gains muscle and power by fueling his body with healthy foods and plenty of exercise.

Regie is made possible in part because of the United Way for Southeastern Michigan and Social Innovation Fund initiative to raise kindergarten readiness from current rates—as low as 14 percent—to 80 percent by 2018.

The NKFM was founded in 1955 with the mission of preventing kidney disease and improving the quality of life for those living with it. Kidney disease is a major health concern because the symptoms of kidney disease are often not detected until the kidneys have lost or decreased function to such a level that life-sustaining measures are required. Millions of people with kidney disease are unaware of it and are not taking the necessary steps to protect their kidneys.

This book is a great way to learn firsthand how Regie's Rainbow Adventure is changing the lives of preschoolers, their families, childcare centers and communities. Children in these programs learn and adopt nutritional and physically active behaviors that prevent chronic disease, promote well-being and ultimately place them on a path to join a generation of healthy, prepared learners.

Enjoy!

Daniel Carney *has been with the National Kidney Foundation of Michigan for 40 years and has served as president and CEO for 30 years.*

Linda Smith-Wheelock *is chief operating officer and executive vice president for the National Kidney Foundation of Michigan.*

Our Story

Did you ever want to be a superhero?

Perhaps you grew up with Superman and Batman. Or perhaps you enjoyed the Teenage Mutant Ninja Turtles, Power Rangers, X-Men, Pokémon, Powerpuff Girls or Spider-Man.

That's a fun question, but it isn't entirely kids' stuff anymore. Superheroes are big business, with the potential to turn the tides of public preference from buying habits to lifestyle choices. Just how hot are superheroes? As of 2016, more than half of the 20 top-grossing Hollywood movies of all time involve superheroes created by Marvel, DC Comics, Disney and other media giants.

The world loves superheroes. Of course, figures with extreme abilities—Samson, Ganesh, Achilles, Robin Hood, Zorro—are as old as civilization. But the tidal wave of popularity we're seeing today is only about a century old. Our current term, "superhero," didn't appear until World War I: That term wasn't widely used until Superman hit newspaper comic strips in the late 1930s. After World War II, however, parents were skeptical of or downright hostile toward these comic characters. In fact, superheroes didn't become a nationally accepted pastime for most kids until the 1970s; those fun-loving Turtles and the noble Power Rangers didn't become a rage until the late 1980s and early 1990s. Pokémon, a franchise now enjoyed by people of all ages on their handheld devices, didn't debut until 1995. The universal celebration of superheroes—nearly every kid's fantasy in some form—is only a couple of decades old.

Today, countless individuals and organizations dream of launching a superhero to catch the public eye and inspire people of all ages to help make the world a better place. But it turns out that this isn't a job most mortals can tackle successfully. For every superhero that truly takes to the skies, countless would-be characters flop. For example: How many of us even remember Izzy, the bug-eyed blue mascot of the 1996 Atlanta Olympics?

This book is the story of one regional nonprofit organization—concerned with the dangerous rise of diabetes and kidney disease across America—whose talented team members have successfully launched a superhero with a bright, healthy future. Most importantly, the National Kidney Foundation of Michigan's "Regie" has successfully withstood the test of thousands of kids who now love this caped, masked, broccoli-shaped superhero! Kids can't wait to tell their parents about their adventures on Regie's colorful islands.

Perhaps most compelling is the fact that rigorous research on Regie's impact indicates that the green guy is doing real work—and getting real results. The Centers for Disease Control and Prevention reports that 93 percent of children in the U.S. do not eat the recommended daily servings of vegetables; 60 percent do not eat the recommended daily servings of fruit. Parents and teachers report increased fruit and vegetable consumption, decreased screen time and increased physical activity as part of the program.

Up! Up and Away! A Morning With Regie

Visitors can't miss the big, green superhero when they walk through the doors of the preschool center run by the New St. Paul Tabernacle Head Start Agency, Inc.

Regie's almost-life-size image hangs on the wall in the main hallway, greeting a group of parents and community leaders who are, on one particular day, paying a visit to the classrooms where teachers are using the National Kidney Foundation of Michigan (NKFM) curriculum. On a table in front of the big Regie poster are handouts for parents, among which are healthy-eating tip sheets produced by the U.S. Department of Agriculture's MyPlate program. This Head Start center is located in a low-income neighborhood, and the nutrition tips are practical both in terms of food preparation and cost. One tip points out that the

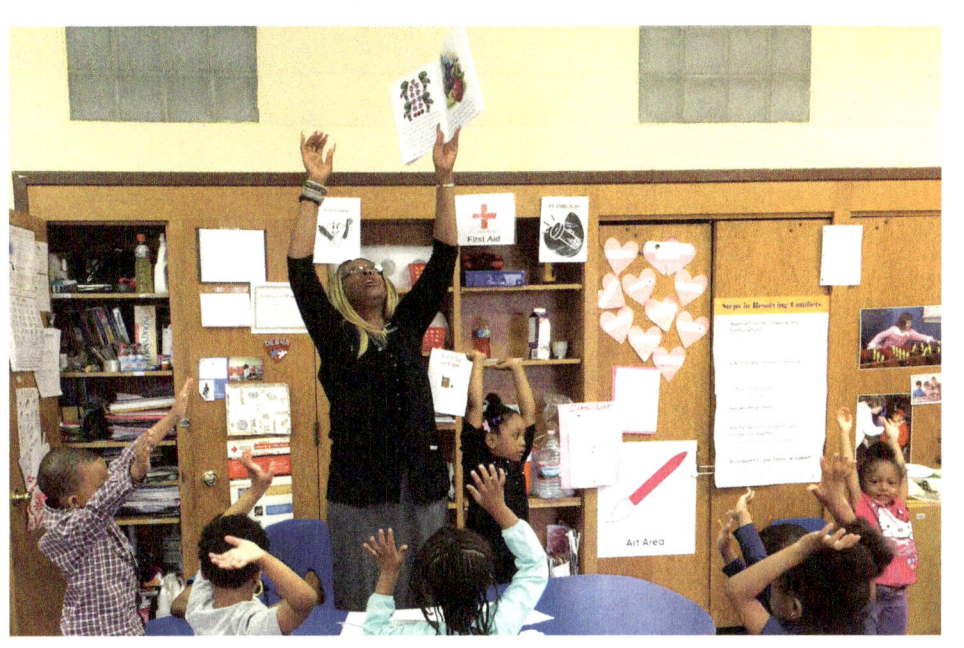

In her classroom at the New St. Paul Tabernacle Head Start Agency in Detroit, Debra Foreman reads a book about Regie's adventures on the Island of Purple. Because the program encourages physical activity, she leads the class in stretching up, into the sky—like their broccoli-shaped superhero.

average prepackaged meal, such as a frozen dinner, costs substantially more than that same meal prepared from scratch. The next tip acknowledges that home cooking takes time and recommends preparing a big batch of food that, once cooked, can be portioned for future meals and frozen. Or, if parents want to try dishes that will add to their family's consumption of vegetables, there are recipes from the NKFM, as well. One full-color recipe sheet shows how to make a batch of Confetti Corn Salsa by combining corn, red or black beans, tomatoes and peppers. The recipe sheet provides two methods of preparation: one involving fresh produce, and another adapted for parents who might not have access to fresh-picked vegetables and need to use canned goods instead. This flexible recipe concept is part of the larger Regie campaign that encourages healthy eating throughout the community.

On this particular day, members of the team that prepared this book arrive at the Head Start center, joining other visitors who catch a glimpse of the superhero's adventures unfolding in the classrooms. When most of the visitors already have chosen other rooms in the building, a few slip into the back of the class run by veteran teacher Debra Foreman. The Regie curriculum is designed to last less than an hour during the Head Start day, once each week, though the specific length of the sessions varies by teacher preference—and "Ms. Foreman," as her name is in the classroom, is known throughout the school for her creativity in bringing Regie to life.

In this classroom, the caped hero's presence is inescapable! A Regie poster hangs on one classroom wall, and a big Regie chart with rainbow-hued rows allows students to line up their own stickers to proudly let the class know they've participated in the Regie program. Finally, there's a poster that shows all of Regie's colorful islands—and is complete with a Regie figure that the teacher can move onto each week's featured island. This week, Regie has been moved to the Island of Purple.

Ms. Foreman teaches a dozen children, with the help of a teaching assistant, in a room organized into specialized areas for play, quiet time, circle sessions, lessons, and arts and crafts. The walls are honeycombed with books, supplies and displays of children's work. When it's time for Regie, Ms. Foreman directs the children to circle around two kidney-shaped tables. She sits at the curved center of one table, surrounded by six children, and directs the lesson for the entire class. Her teaching assistant sits with the other six children at the second table.

"Now, let's all sit down in our chairs!" Ms. Foreman calls, her voice warm yet loud enough to slice through the murmuring of a dozen children moving around and chattering with one another. "I'm going to read our Regie story! We're going to read! So take your seats. We want to meet Regie this week! It's Regie time! Please sit down!"

One boy flips his chair backward and straddles it.

"Is that how we sit in our chairs? No it isn't. But you know that, don't you? How do we sit? You can show me, can't you?"

Ms. Foreman says, continuing her pointed instructions to the boy until he dutifully turns his chair the correct way and sits politely. She shifts the message to one of encouragement.

"That's right! That's how we sit."

She calls to the entire class, "The big question today: What island are we going to visit with Regie?" The answer is in her hand as she waves one of the seven Regie story books toward the children.

"Purple! Purple!" children begin to shout, settling into their chairs as their eyes land on the big, bright book Ms. Foreman is waving.

"You're right. Yes, you are. Purple. And before I read today's story … " Ms. Foreman says, pausing to bring out a gallon-sized plastic bag of fruit. "Before we read, can someone tell me: What are these? We're going to taste these today. What are these? What's in my hand, here?"

A dozen sets of young eyes shift to the bag in the teacher's hand. The murmur rises to a low roar until someone finally shouts, clearly, "Apples!"

Ms. Foreman smiles. "*Are* these apples? What *are* these? Look closely. What's in my hand, right here?"

Finally, someone says, "Purple plums!"

"That's right!" she says. "These are purple plums because we are traveling to what island?" And she shifts to display the hand holding the book again.

"The Island of Purple!" someone shouts.

"Are we ready to take our adventure?" she asks. The young voices are at a low roar, but as she motions for quiet and settles into her own seat, that noise falls back to a murmur. Then, the room becomes almost quiet. "Everybody ready for me to read, now?" she asks. "Everybody listening? Eyes right here. We want to meet Regie, don't we?"

"**Yeaaaah!**" the kids at her table shout back.

She leans toward the other table, where the six children did not respond as enthusiastically. "And my children at the other table? Are you ready for me to read? Can you show me you're ready? Are you sitting in your chairs? OK. OK, now. Are you ready for me to read?"

"**Yeaaah!**" the kids at the other table respond.

The seven Regie books are short. There are only seven pages of illustrations and accompanying text in the Island of Purple book. The books are large in size, with vivid pictures contrasted by bright-white backgrounds. Every child can clearly see what's happening on each page of the story.

In Ms. Foreman's classroom, all eyes are locked on the first page as Ms. Foreman reads about Regie arriving on the Island of Purple to meet Señor Cabbage, Ms. Plum and Ms. Purple Fig. As she turns the pages, she pauses to discuss several pictures, asking children to identify fruits, vegetables and other elements they see on the pages—including the roller skates worn by one friendly, fruit-shaped character. Then she pauses her storytelling, briefly responding to a boy who has just stood up and decided to wander away from the group. It takes just a few moments of Ms. Foreman's "laser" eye and commanding voice to bring him back to his chair. While corralling the wayward boy, she barely misses a beat in Regie's adventure. Next, she reaches a page specially designed for counting. With the class, she counts out nine purple cabbages and three plums. Ms. Foreman then points out number symbols elsewhere on the page, connecting the number symbols to the act of counting. She goes back and forth with children on this counting exercise.

Pointing to the three plums on the page, Ms. Foreman asks, "And what about these plums right here? We are going to taste plums today. So let's be thinking about: What happens if I eat a plum? What does that make me?"

"It makes you strong!" shouts a girl.

"Yes, it makes us strong! And what else? What else does eating our fruit help us with?"

"Memory!" someone cries.

"Yes, it does. It helps our memory. And what else? There's more! The most important thing to remember is—and say this with me: It makes me feel good inside!"

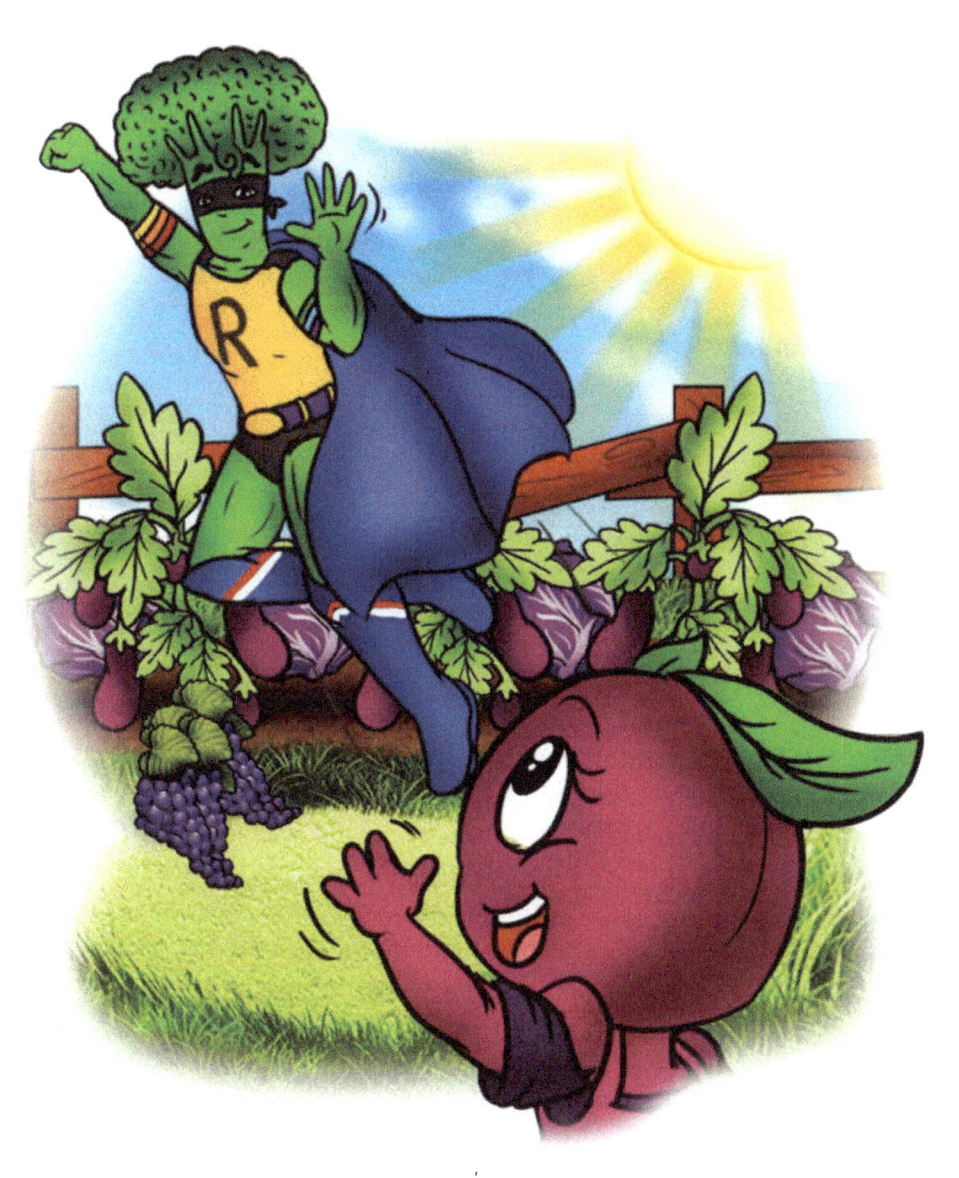

The power Regie felt he just couldn't believe.

"Please give me my purple stripe before I must leave.

A page from the Island of Purple book as the superhero bids farewell to Ms. Plum.

She repeats that line again, slowly now, and everyone chimes in on the phrase, "Feeeel gooood insiiiiide."

The final page of each book contains a riddle, so Ms. Foreman says, "Now it's time for our riddle this week! It's time for our riddle. This is our purple riddle: 'I'm purple and round. I look like a ball. I'll help with your memory. My pit is real small. What am I?'"

Several children shout, "A purple plum!"

"Yes! That's right. I'm a purple plum. And that's what we're going to taste today! But before we do that, can you remember the other islands we've visited with Regie? Can you remember our other riddles? Here's one: 'I grow on a tree and people say if you eat me, you'll keep the doctor away. My color is red. What am I?'"

"You're a strawberry!" cries a boy.

"No, I'm not a strawberry in this riddle. But you know, that's a good guess. Strawberries are red and they're good for us, too. What am I in this riddle—one of me a day keeps the doctor away? And I'm red."

"Apple!" says a girl.

"That's right!" Ms. Foreman reviews other colors and has the children make up their own riddles, some of which are more challenging than others. One girl gets nervous as she tries to announce her riddle to the class and blurts out, "I'm a plum! What am I?" So the class talks about riddles and how to make a riddle. That little girl gets another chance and manages, this time, to say, "I'm blue and I'm good for you! And I'm a berry. What am I?"

"Yes, now that's a better riddle. Yes, it is. I wonder what she is. Class?"

Someone yells, "You're a blueberry!" At that, the little girl looks very pleased: she laughs, and stands, and twirls around. This behavior prompts restlessness in other children, and the room's general murmur is rising to a roar again when Ms. Foreman chooses this moment to have the class practice their superhero moves. She stands up abruptly and calls the children to "Reach up with me now! Reach up your arms very high, like

Regie taking off! Can you stretch like Regie?" She maintains a constant narration until all 12 children are on their feet with her, all reaching toward the ceiling.

"And can we stretch from side to side?" she asks, coaching them along. "Side to side, now! Like Regie, twisting and turning. Like Regie! Yes! Yes! Ohhhh, can you just feel all the energy that we are getting as we stretch? We're feeling strong inside! When we are active, you know, we feel so good inside, don't we? Let's move! Move!" And the Regie exercises continue for several minutes. While the class is moving in sync with her, Ms. Foreman concludes that they're ready to sit again.

Finally, it's time to taste the plums.

"Hands on laps as we sit in our chairs! Hands on laps as we sit in our chairs!" Ms. Foreman chants. "Hands on laps! Hands on laps!" Now that the children are seated, and not leaning onto the two tables, Ms. Foreman can move around the room to wipe the tabletops with a cleanser and pull on plastic gloves to handle the fruit.

As she holds up a plum, Ms. Foreman asks an important question.

"So, what do you think we will find inside this fruit?"

A few of the children seem to be familiar with plums, but many of the children appear to have never seen the whole, unpeeled fruits introduced in various Regie sessions. In an earlier week, a fresh pineapple had completely stumped the kids.

"What is inside this purple plum? Will it be purple inside, like the skin of the fruit?"

Some heads nod; some heads shake back and forth.

"What will the color be inside this plum? And what will it taste like? That's the question now! And I want you to make a prediction: Can you say if this fruit will be sweet or sour? Tangy? Bitter?"

"Sour!" shouts a boy.

"That is your prediction. He is thinking about this plum and he is anticipating that the fruit will be sour inside, once I cut it open. Does that sound right? Any other predictions?"

Ms. Foreman keeps this line of questioning going until she has seen each child take a good look at the plum and has heard each one respond. Nearly all of them pick from her choice of four terms. Only one boy varies, and says, "I think it will taste like an orange."

"Now, that's a different prediction! I like oranges, too," says Ms. Foreman. "So, you think it will taste like an orange. That's a very interesting guess. OK, then, it's time to taste our fruit and see if our predictions were correct." And she turns to a girl sitting to her left, who has been appointed helper for the day. "Michai, it's time to give each person a plate. Everyone needs their own plate so I can give you each a piece of this plum to taste."

Michai hops to her feet, walks to a cupboard, gathers the small plates and distributes them around the tables.

"While Michai does that, we'll clean our hands. Clean our hands. Clean our hands." Ms. Foreman keeps chanting as she produces wipes and goes to work, watching as each child uses a wipe. "OK, now what did we just do? We wiped our table. We keep our work area clean when we work with food, don't we? We cleaned our hands. Now, we're going to taste."

The first boy who samples a crescent of plum exclaims, "Sweeeet! It's sweet."

"Yes it is," Ms. Foreman says. "These are really sweet plums today."

The next boy drops it onto his plate without tasting it and turns away from her.

"Remember our rule? Remember? We take a taste, don't we?"

He nods, picks it up, and takes a bite.

"Sour," he says, shaking his head.

"Well, now, that's true, too! These plums are very sweet, but they're also a little sour, aren't they?"

A girl starts chanting, "A little bit of sour makes it taste so sweet! A little bit of sour makes it taste so sweet!" Ms. Foreman picks up that chant and keeps it going. Finally, Ms. Foreman has gone all the way around the circle and has returned to her helper, Michai, age 5. This young helper makes a great display of accepting the last crescent of plum and taking a big bite. She nods her head thoughtfully as she tastes it. She makes a sound.

"Michai, what did you say to describe the taste?"

"I didn't say nothing," Michai says, still chewing.

"You mean you did not say *anything*," Ms. Foreman corrects. "So, you are still eating. I see that. I'll let you finish. We'll let everyone finish the plum now. And now? Now, we're all finished. So, Michai, what do you say about it?"

"I say they're really sweet," Michai says. And then she declares, "They are so sweet that I believe I've got a song about this plum."

"You have a song?" Ms. Foreman says, her eyebrows raised. "You've made up a song. OK. OK. Yes, to finish our tasting today, I think we should hear that song." She looks down at Michai again to be sure. "You've got a song, right? You've made up a song about the plum?"

Michai is nodding proudly. She's ready. She sings in a bouncy melody:

"There's a little young plum going up the street!
That little young plum's coming right to me!
Then, God looks down and sees it go!
And God feels very happy."

Then, in a deep, booming voice, Michai adds as if from above:

"Go, Ms. Plum! Go! Go! Go!"

"There's more!" she tells Ms. Foreman. Her bouncy melody ends with a refrain:

"That's why my plum tastes sweet, sweet, sweet!
And God is very happy!"

And, there is more. The children get stickers because they have participated in the program, and they are able to place these stickers on the big classroom chart that shows their progress with tasting new foods.

In Ms. Foreman's classroom, traveling with Regie over a series of weeks also involves making colorful little passports with construction-paper covers and white pages. The children decorate their passports with pictures of the fruits and vegetables

Our Story • 15

they have tasted. So, as the tasting portion of the morning ends, there's a whirlwind of activity as children place their stickers and take their passports to their individual storage bins. One little girl pauses to tell Ms. Foreman that she plans to present her passport to her mother, so they can revisit all of the islands together.

"So, you'll be going on an adventure with Regie together!" Ms. Foreman says.

The girl nods, smiling broadly.

"My mom's going to like this. She likes good food."

Confronting the Challenge in Childhood

Linda Smith-Wheelock is chief operating officer and executive vice president for the National Kidney Foundation of Michigan (NKFM) and has worked with the nonprofit for more than two decades. This is her story:

I had worked with community mental health programs before deciding to join the National Kidney Foundation of Michigan, and what attracted me to this organization was its openness to innovation. The level of excitement and commitment among the staff about the importance of the work they were doing together was invigorating.

Regie has been evolving over the past decade, but the foundations of this work go back much further. In the mid 1990s, our team at the NKFM was working with professionals from state government—what today is the Michigan Department of Health and Human Services—and focusing on public health and the prevention of kidney disease. At that time, we were talking about ways to be more "upfront" in our strategy for addressing chronic disease. To us, that phrase really meant that we needed to work more with children on health and wellness in order to get out in front of the disease. Now, years later, we have compiled a lot of research on the rising obesity rates among American children—as well as the causes and effects of this

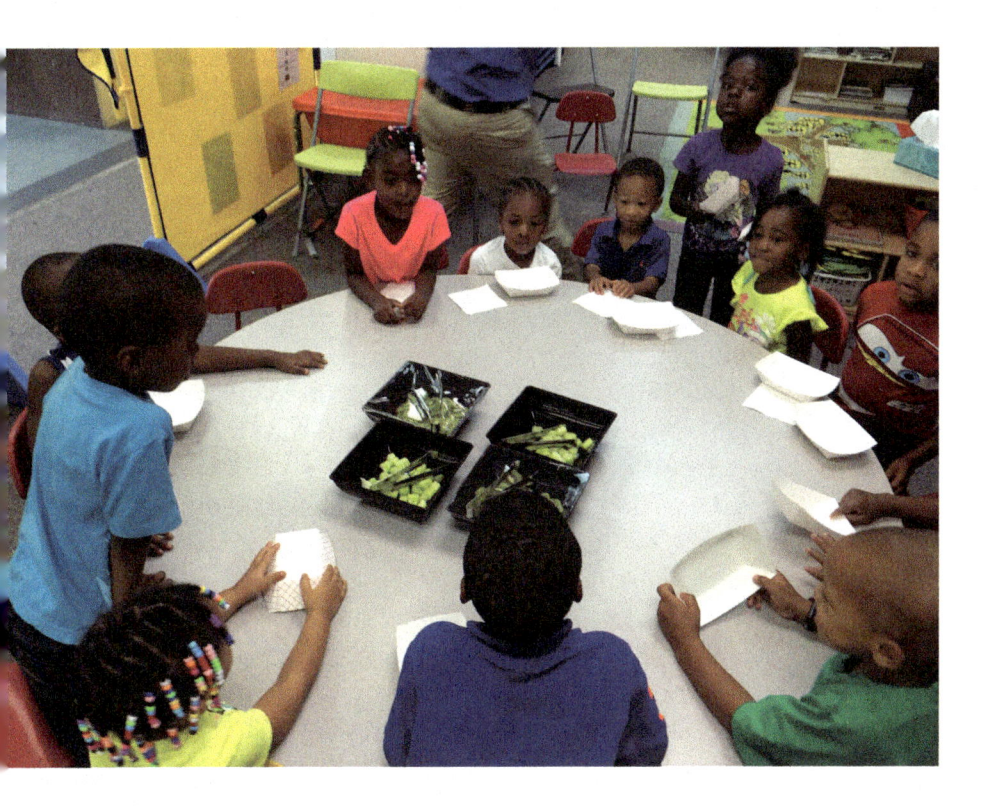

Children eager to taste samples from Regie's Island of Green.

problem. But even in the 1990s, without all of the studies we have today, it was becoming clear that we needed to work with children on health and wellness. One reason we began looking at this age was that early research showed that children could help their parents adopt healthier eating habits; the most effective time to reach adults on these issues is in the period when parents are already making changes in the home because of their children's needs and preferences. Parents have a strong incentive to make changes when they know their children will grow up stronger and healthier as a result.

We are very encouraged today by the body of data showing the effectiveness of our Regie program. Of course, now, there are many efforts all across the country to address these issues with children, including Michelle Obama's Let's Move! public health campaign. I hope readers of our book will be inspired to learn more about this, and perhaps to join this movement. Information is now available from a wide variety of public sources, including the Centers for Disease Control and Prevention and the Let's Move! website, which in itself is co-sponsored by a half-dozen federal agencies: http://www.letsmove.gov/

Here is a quick summary from Let's Move!:

The Let's Move! campaign was founded on the understanding that childhood obesity rates have increased exponentially in the past three decades. Thirty years ago, children got more daily exercise and ate healthier meals. Now, with the average family facing increased demands on their time, families eat fewer home-cooked meals and don't get the daily-recommended amount of exercise. Because of this, many children are qualified as obese, and face many future health problems because of this.

Even though we now know this trend started in the 1980s, it took a while for us to reach a national consensus on the problem—and for research to show us the best ways to address the challenge. Our agency was working on this in the 1990s and early 2000s, and by 2005, our NKFM strategic plan was to emphasize the importance of work with children in pre-K to 12th grade. To reach that level of focused concern took us a while. But, by 2005, the National Kidney Foundation of Michigan was publishing clear recommendations, including the following:

> American children eat more and exercise less than ever before. Computers, TV and video games, combined with cheap, high-caloric food, have taken a serious toll on the health of an entire generation…. Socially and emotionally, obese children rate their quality of life lower than normal-weight children. Physically, they experience the same risk factors associated with heart disease in adults: high cholesterol, hypertension and type 2 diabetes. Our recommendation: Work with stakeholders within Michigan to create a demonstration project focusing on policy, environmental and behavioral changes

and designed to reduce the number of community members at risk for chronic kidney disease. The ultimate goal: Influence at-risk individuals to adopt healthier lifestyles, one community at a time.

Originally, we had started working in schools with a program called Kids Interested in the Care of Kidneys—a program focused on high school students. It was based on materials from another kidney foundation, which we got permission to use. The goal was to teach kids about the importance of their kidneys and how kidney disease could affect their lives. We provided this educational program to teachers and hoped that they would use our lesson plans.

All of that was before we thought of focusing on younger children. At that time, in Michigan, the NKFM worked with a program called the Michigan Diabetes Outreach Network, in connection with the State of Michigan and the Centers for Disease Control and Prevention. At first, we worked with two of the regional networks—one of them in the Detroit area and another one in the Flint area. Eventually, we started working with a third network, in the Grand Rapids area. Through these partnerships, we had nurses and dietitians on staff who would visit schools to help kids who had juvenile or type 1 diabetes. In these visits, they would also educate teachers and other school personnel about caring for diabetes. Through these programs, our team developed additional resources and worked with health-care systems throughout the region to promote education and better self-regulation for people living with diabetes.

The opportunity to reach people through prevention efforts is powerful, and the NKFM has been fortunate to have many experiences in doing so. Our first prevention-based initiative was launched in 1999 and was called "Healthy Hair Starts With a Healthy Body." Diabetes is more prevalent in the African-American community and we felt it was crucial that we develop a prevention program that was accessible to members of this community. We found that some of the most trusted figures in African-American communities are hairstylists who regularly consult with their clients. So we started training African-American hairstylists so that they could discuss nutrition and healthy activity—both chronic disease preventatives—with their clients. The stylists encouraged their clients to make health-behavior changes like increasing their consumption of fruits and vegetables; switching to nonfat or low-fat foods; increasing their physical activity; or visiting a doctor for a checkup. Connecting with a trusted figure within the community was successful, and ended up supporting our Regie's Rainbow Adventure® program model that we created later on.

Making wise decisions with the funds entrusted to us is one of our core values—and that's why we are always looking for evidence of each program's effectiveness. In 2016, the National Kidney Foundation of Michigan received a four out of a four-star rating from the national charity watchdog organization, Charity Navigator—for the ninth consecutive year. Scoring 98.5 out of 100 total points, NKFM is in the upper 1 percent of all nonprofits in America. The Charity Navigator rating highlights our integrity, reliability, accountability, transparency and fiscal responsibility.

That solid foundation allows us to continue innovating, testing, evaluating—and looking for new partners. When Regie came along, it was natural for us to connect with the Social Innovation Fund through United Way for Southeastern Michigan. As of autumn 2016, Regie's Rainbow Adventure has served 192 preschools, including 157 Head Starts, and has reached a total of 12,588 children.

Arthur Franke, Ph.D., is senior vice president and chief science officer for the National Kidney Foundation of Michigan. This is his story:

How did Regie become a part of our programming? Here is the progression that led to Regie's arrival:

Since we were founded in 1955, our mission has always been to prevent kidney disease and to improve the quality of life for those who have it. A major priority within that mission is preventing people from ever reaching the point of kidney failure.

The leading cause of kidney failure is uncontrolled diabetes; and the second cause is uncontrolled high blood pressure. We address the causes of these conditions by encouraging healthier eating and more physical activity. And we know that we especially need to address these issues in communities where there is disproportionate risk. People of color are four to five times more likely to develop kidney disease when compared with the population as a whole. In short, that's why we develop the kinds of programs we've launched through the years—and that's why we eventually launched Regie. Along the way, it's the reason why we decided to work with hairstylists and, later, to add Dodge the Punch to train African-American barbers, as well.

These programs work. People like them. Awareness helps people make a difference in their lives. One of the most difficult parts of this kind of work is that people don't physically feel bad as they are developing diabetes or high blood pressure. Unless they're going to a doctor on a regular basis, they may not even be aware that they have these conditions. We know that 75 percent of cases of kidney failure could have been prevented—so awareness can make a huge difference.

I oversee our prevention programs, which we know are very effective and cost saving. And as I say that, I want to stress: We use evidence-based programs, meaning that we've got solid research showing us that these things we're doing are effective. That's why what we are doing today took so long to develop. As Linda Smith-Wheelock has explained, it took years for the data to tell us that obesity was becoming such a crucial problem nationwide. We know now that this trend toward obesity has been growing gradually for several decades—but research and reporting took a while to catch up. Even as the evidence was showing us that children were struggling with these issues, we did not immediately have evidence-based programming that we could use to prevent children from becoming overweight. It's a very complex problem that grew over many years and bending the curve of this national trend is a challenge that didn't come with a quick fix.

We did realize that we needed to work with children, but we reached out to middle schools and high schools first. We also knew that we would need innovative approaches if we were going to engage young people. That was the overall context and concept when the NKFM office in Flint, which was housed in a YMCA building, told us about a day camp that its employees were organizing. For one week, kids would come to the YMCA daily; the nonprofit was interested in including a nutrition-based program as part of each day. Team members in that office came up with an idea with a rainbow theme, designed for kids age 6 and under, that would encourage trying fruits and vegetables in the colors of the rainbow. That ended up working out very well, so we also used this idea in the Pontiac area. That was where the seeds for Regie were planted. We got great feedback from the children and their families on the theme of "eating the rainbow," and the Regie figure came to the forefront as the symbol and storyline that tied the whole program together. At first, in Flint and Pontiac, we were just getting this anecdotal evidence from people involved in those programs—but it was very positive. Head Start programs began showing interest so we decided to expand. We eventually got many people involved in refining the program and developing the superhero who brought it all to life in such a memorable way for the children.

So, even before the Social Innovation Fund (SIF) grant came along, we had the beginnings of a fun program that teachers liked, children enjoyed and parents praised. It was even becoming a success in some of the Oakland Livingston Human Service Agency Head Start programs, northwest of the Detroit area. We wanted to touch more lives with the program and we knew that this growth could be very helpful to Head Starts in Detroit and Wayne County.

This set us up to actually apply for the SIF grant on behalf of the National Kidney Foundation of Michigan. Our goal was to ramp up what became known as Regie's Rainbow Adventure and to reach thousands of kids with Regie's message. We also began working with the University of Michigan School of Public Health to build the base of evidence that confirmed the impact of Regie. As always, we want to see if there is solid evidence of the program's effectiveness and, while the entire study is incomplete at the time this book was published, the preliminary data looks quite positive. Parents are telling us, "My kids are now eating fruits and vegetables they never wanted to try before." They tell us it's because Regie wants kids to become strong. We also try to reduce what we call "screen time." We want kids to realize that they need to incorporate physical activity into their day and not just stare at computer or game or TV screens. And that effort seems to be working, as well.

Teachers like the Regie program because it comes to them with a complete curriculum they can use, including all of the colorful books and posters. The lessons allow teachers to use lots of different options, depending on their individual classroom goals. There are opportunities to exercise skills with numbers, in counting and with colors—and connections with math and science, as well. Regie also promotes physical activity, which teachers can link to their goals in the classroom.

Here's the basic description: Regie's Rainbow Adventure is a seven-week program implemented by teachers who are trained by our NKFM staff. Teachers are presented with the program's purpose, an implementation timeline, and a thorough explanation on how to use the program's materials. Teachers are also provided with a step-by-step, best practice curriculum that details the steps of program implementation.

Our program coordinators make phone and email contacts throughout the implementation to receive programming updates and provide guidance and support as needed. We consider the heart of this program to be the series of storybooks, the weekly food-tasting sessions and the weekly outreach to parents. In addition to getting kids excited about nutrition, each book incorporates important child development skills like counting, color identification, new vocabulary and learning through movement.

The Regie Bag

Each year, we provide teachers with the materials they need to welcome Regie. Currently, our resource bags include the following:

- **Teacher's manual**—Our manual was developed to provide teachers with step-by-step guidance on how to successfully present Regie's Rainbow Adventure®. The manual describes the program, explains how to introduce Regie in the classroom, how the island theme unfolds and how to plan each week's lesson. For new teachers, our complete training includes a detailed orientation to the teacher's manual. Returning teachers are familiar with the program, so we instead focus on any updates or fresh ideas.
- **Regie books**—Colorful Regie books carry classes through the seven-week program. We offer a complete set of these books to teachers each year.
- **Island poster**—The 11-by-17-inch island poster is a great tool to use when introducing Regie to students. The poster includes an introductory message and also a small Regie image that teachers can cut out, so that children can move "Regie" around the islands as the class visits each one.
- **Regie poster**—The 11-by-17-inch Regie poster shows Regie gaining his power stripes as he actively completes his visits and eats his fruits and vegetables. On the poster, Regie's power stripes are white, so each week, students can fill in the stripes with that week's color.
- **Name chart**—The 11-by-17-inch name chart is rainbow-colored and shows the children progressing through their adventures with Regie. Each child's name is written on the chart, and the children place stickers every week to show that they have completed another part of the journey with Regie.
- **Parent handouts**—Each week, parents receive a one-page handout that explains the theme of the week,

summarizes the week's story, shows examples of fruits and vegetables in that week's color and offers a fun-and-easy recipe to try at home. These handouts help parents to enjoy the adventures with their children as they talk at home and sample more of the new foods the children tasted in class.

- **Surveys**—At the end of the seven-week program, surveys are distributed to parents and teachers so that we can receive feedback on our programming.
- **Fruit and vegetable cards**—The 3 ½- by-4 ½-inch fruit and vegetable cards provide many options for classroom use. The entire set displays three fruits or vegetables for each color in the program. We give teachers two sets of the cards, so that teachers can use them to play a matching game. They also can be used as flash cards. The words on the cards are in both English and Spanish.

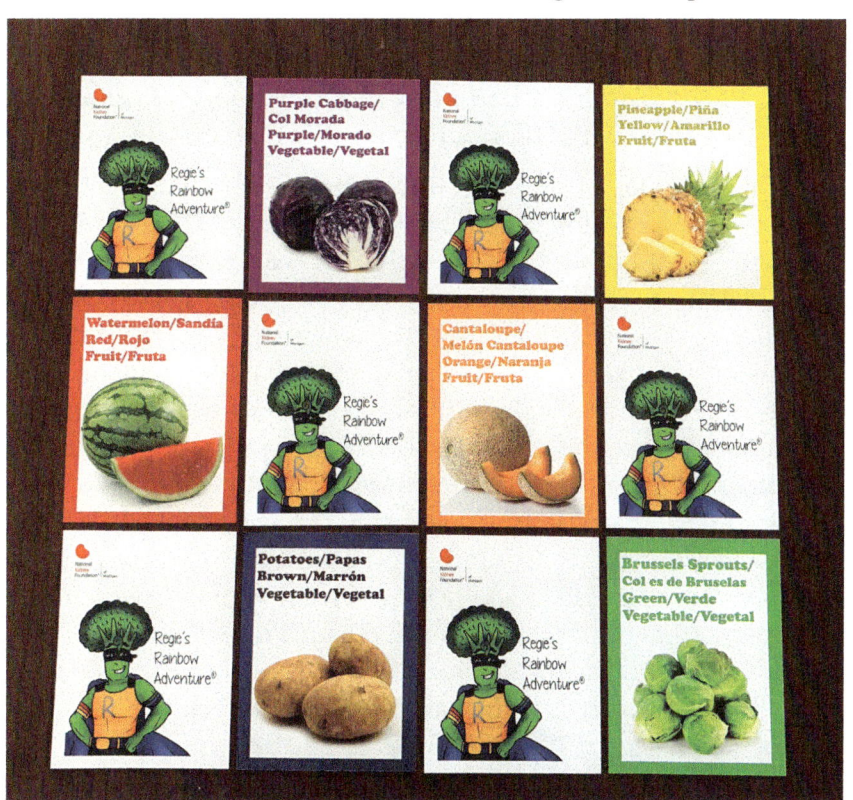

Samples of the colorful Regie fruit and vegetable cards, with text in English and Spanish.

Why does the Regie program work? It's fun. Kids get to engage with a superhero who looks like a big stalk of broccoli! That's an idea that makes anyone smile—and makes you want to find out more about this unusual superhero. Regie's success ultimately comes down to that one word: fun.

It's very hard to confront the upward trend in childhood obesity, as it is so widespread and has built up over so many years. But we are seeing evidence emerge that this kind of program eventually will help us to bend the curve on that trend.

Regie Comes to Life

Paul and Stephanie Zafarana run Pica Marketing Group, the southeast Michigan company that helped the National Kidney Foundation of Michigan design the Regie puppet. Over the decades, Pica has designed a huge array of promotional products—from hats to backpacks, board games to stuffed animals—and now, the Regie puppet ranks among their most popular efforts. This is Paul's story:

Initially, one of our healthcare clients made the connection between our company and the National Kidney Foundation of Michigan. This was back when the NKFM was first developing Regie and before they got the federal grant to expand the program. When we met, I saw the potential right away. I'm a dad with two kids, so I know the demographic for this personally; I also knew how powerful this could be if we asked the right questions while this project was still in the early stages of development. One of the first questions we discussed was: How do you engage this market with a figure who will interest kids from a wide range of backgrounds? You need a figure who will appeal to everyone and isn't identified specifically with one particular group of people. So I really liked the idea of working with a figure shaped like a stalk of broccoli

Next, we agreed on the basic outcomes we wanted and on our call to action: **We want kids to explore fruits and**

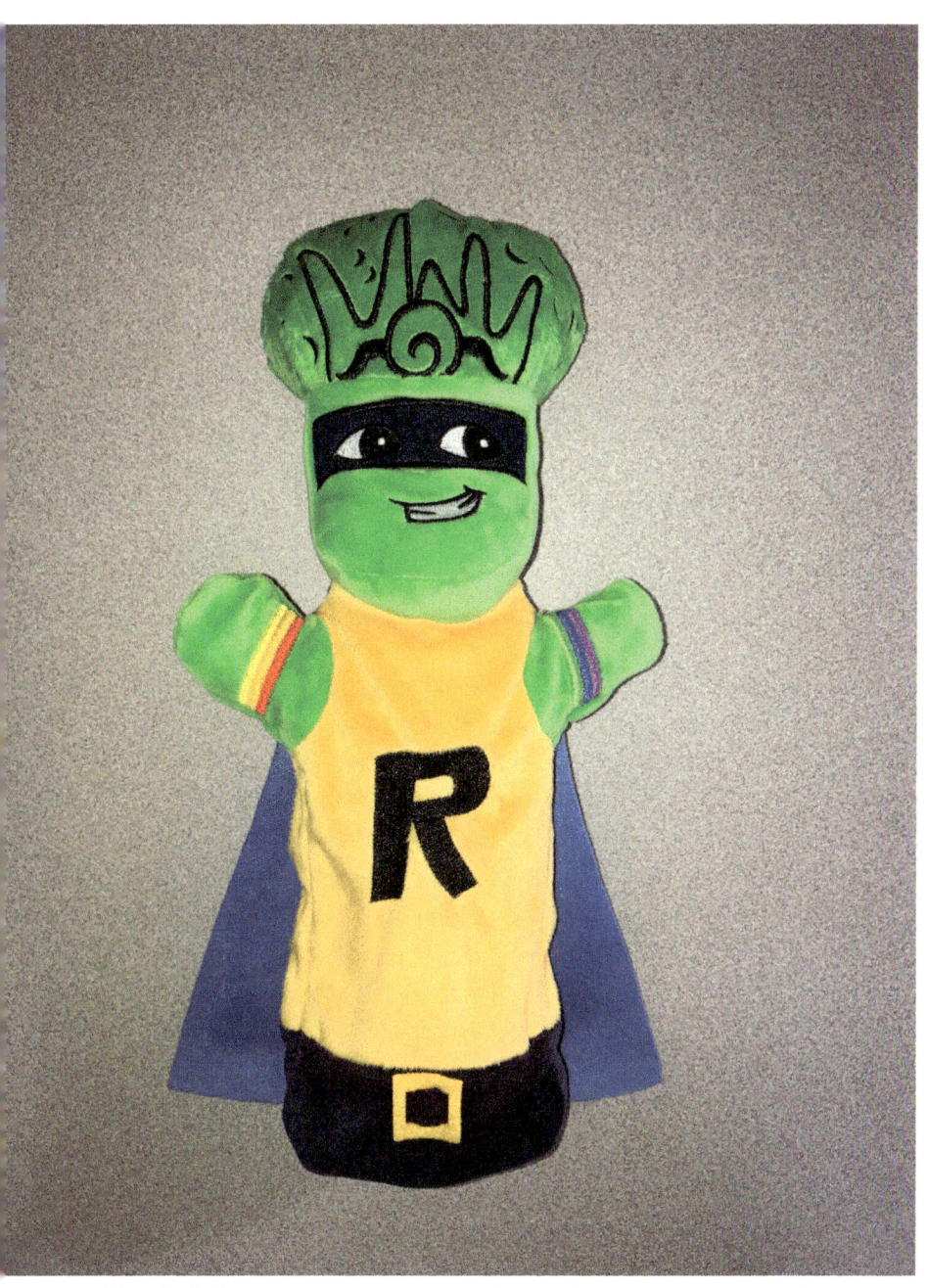

The plush Regie puppet is one option for teachers to use to present the program, while telling stories or introducing fruits and vegetables.

Our Story • 27

vegetables and wind up eating more of them—and we want the kids to convince their parents to get involved, too. The challenge for us was to build this around a figure the kids could relate to. That started with lots of sketches of Regie, drawn by kids themselves. Before we were done with that phase, we had numerous images on the table. In developing the final image, we also had some practical concerns: We wanted a design that could be converted into a physical figure. We wanted to make it into a moveable puppet. That's why the broccoli idea was so compelling. We could see how a half-broccoli half-man figure could form and how that could become a physical piece—in our case, a two-dimensional puppet. We wanted that kind of physical presence in the classroom. Then, we decided that we wanted the body of the puppet to be plush because kids of that age really gravitate toward the feel of soft textures. We knew that bringing Regie to life in this way would have a much greater impact than would putting his picture on a pencil or a baseball cap for the kids.

Next, we faced the basic question: Could we pull off this idea? The answer was: Yes. We could easily make a plush puppet. These days, plush figures are a common kind of promotional product, which means it was practical to have them made in quantity at an affordable cost. Our company has a lot of experience working with factories that produce promotional plush products.

As you read this book about Regie—and should you want to jump into this area of promotion for your own group or non-profit—there are a few things I would advise. The first is to make sure you've got your funding secured or your initial expenditures, for scaling up the program and for your ongoing operating costs. You need a solid financial plan.

Second, make sure you're clear about your desired outcomes—your expected return on investment. Ask yourself: Does it make sense to develop promotional materials for the desired response? Will the extra investment in promotion help people to interact with the program that much more? Does it make good business sense to do this? These are just some of the questions you can ask.

Then, don't start the process by insisting on a single, specific kind of promotion. There are so many options out there—TV, radio, direct mail—depending on your budget. The NKFM made some specific choices about Regie in regards to the puppet, the books and the costumes that people wear to make appearances as Regie. After a lot of planning and development, the end result of those choices now brings the program to life and helps the NKFM to get the outcomes desired. But, if you're just starting out, make sure to consider the whole range of options available to your organization.

Other important questions to ask as you begin are: What's your call to action? Why would people want to interact with you? If they do interact with you, what, specifically, do you want them to do as a result? Many people tend to skip right over these questions. But it's very important to develop a clear call to action. If you are clear about these things from the beginning, it's going to make your consultation with marketing professionals much more effective.

What a marketing professional will offer is help with the overall presentation. Think about this: What's the difference between a fast-food burger that costs less than $1 and a high-end restaurant burger that costs more than $10? The major difference is presentation. If you're paying more than $10 for your burger, you're expecting to enjoy a whole set of experiences that come with your much-more-expensive dinner: the premium ingredients, the atmosphere of the restaurant, the enjoyment of being with friends in the setting of that particular restaurant, and so on. The kind of question we ask in marketing is: What are the experiences people are hoping to have when they choose this product or program?

Remember to leave room for revision as you learn from your experience. Most people who already know about Regie may not realize this, but the NKFM continues to improve Regie all the time. In the early planning phase with Regie, I remember that we discussed having two kinds of figures: first, the puppet, and second, a 2-foot-tall plush figure that each school could put in a display case as a constant reminder of the program. But it turned out that the puppet was such a success, we decided to keep focusing on the puppet. Teachers love that they can bring Regie to life by using the puppet in intimate settings with the children circled around them. The puppet is more effective than a stuffed figure for this age range and in these kinds of settings. So, that's one change we made: We never produced the stuffed figure. Now, even the Regie puppet is changing. There's a new version now that's closer to Emily Zieroth's illustrations of the character in the books. It's important to learn from your experience and adapt.

Finally, as you develop your plan, get it all down in writing and make sure your whole team understands the plan. Make sure you can explain it to others, too. A successful outcome for a program as big as Regie's Rainbow Adventure takes lots of dedicated people making it happen in classroom after classroom, year after year. As marketing professionals, we are one cog in the larger engine that makes Regie go and keeps the program expanding.

Emily Zieroth is an illustrator who has worked on dozens of children's books and other illustrated media, from banners to T-shirts to animation. With the Social Innovation Fund, the National Kidney Foundation of Michigan had the resources to revamp its original Regie stories, which had never been professionally illustrated. They selected Emily for the project. This is her story:

When the NKFM contacted me about this project, they explained that they wanted to update the Regie stories, and that I should use the original sketches as an inspiration for my work. I was sent a PDF of the original stories and the Regie text is still the original text—but the stories had never before been published in the quality of paperback format they are today. The NKFM had some of the key ideas already set—like Regie earning his power stripes as he traveled between the islands—but they wanted me to put my own twist and style on this superhero and his adventures.

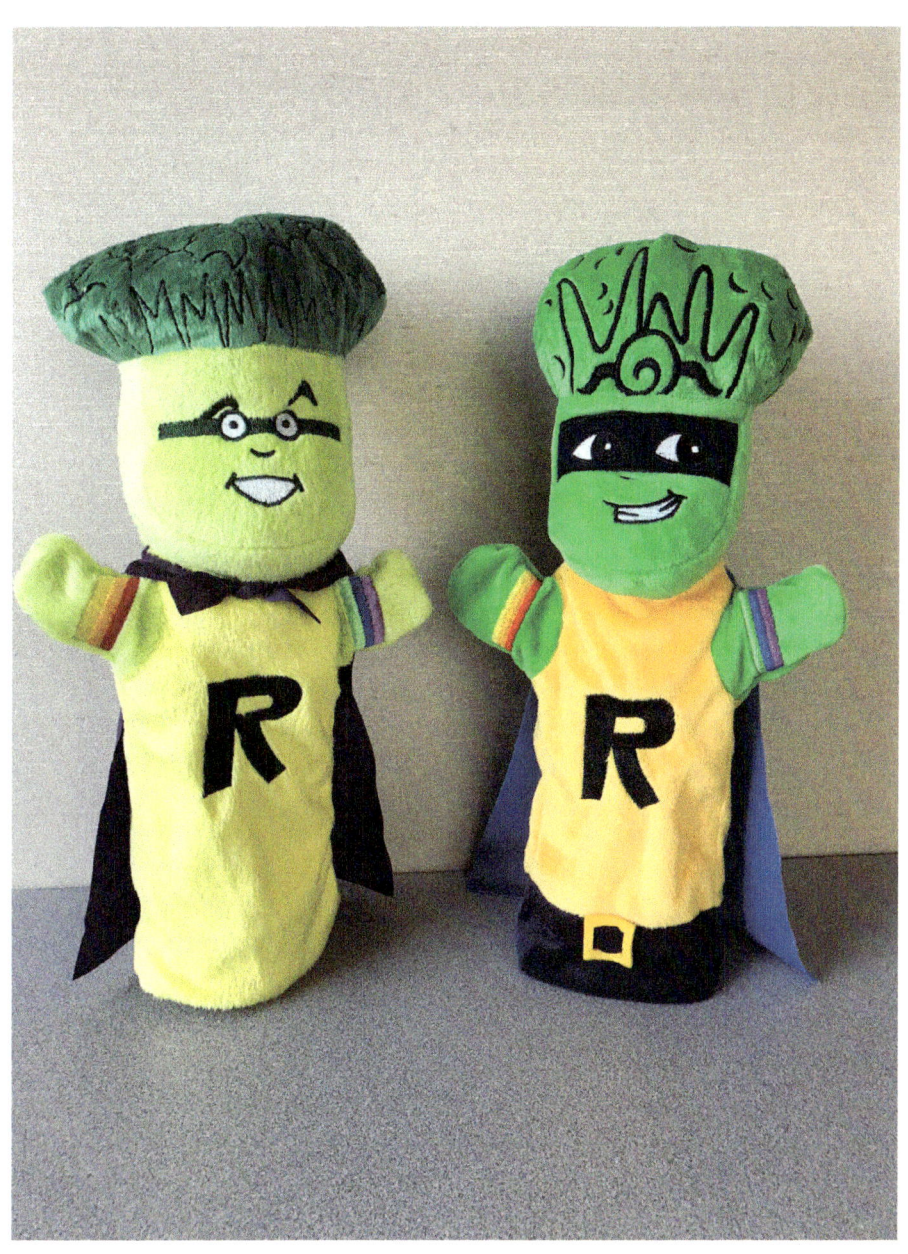

The publication of the seven Regie books, with illustrations by artist Emily Zieroth, led to an updating of the Regie puppet. Today, hundreds of the puppets in both designs are used across Michigan.

Our Story • 31

Over the years, I've illustrated lots of children's books that contain lessons. I've worked on books about sharing, dental care, courage, saving money and other themes. So, this project was a good fit for me.

My own first reaction to Regie was: *Great! It's going to be a fun, creative challenge to draw this broccoli superhero who is teaching people to eat better.* I really enjoyed the work from the start. And I have to say: Regie did affect me. I've always enjoyed my sweets, so spending time living with Regie was a great opportunity for me to think about my own nutrition, even as I was helping the NKFM reach out to kids through the books.

As I had thought from the start, creating these books turned out to be a fun process. I'm very familiar with this kind of illustration, and I love lots of different styles: I like Disney and Don Bluth, who did *All Dogs Go to Heaven* and *American Tail*. I also like Andrew Hou, who is based in Korea and does this amazing series using colorful little figures to tell the ongoing story of his relationship with his wife. So, in envisioning Regie for these new books, I had lots of creative ideas and options in mind. The biggest tension lied in wondering of how to portray Regie so that young children would understand right away that he was a superhero—and they wouldn't be scared of him. Regie had to have an amusing side, even while he was showing off his superpowers. So my first choice was to show him as visibly muscular. He is a superhero, after all. Kids loved the idea that, if they ate their fruits and vegetables and got some physical activity, they could grow up big and strong like Regie. Maybe not as a stalk of broccoli! But, you get the idea. As a nod to the original Superman, I did put a signature green curl at Regie's forehead. The mask I designed gives him, I think, an air of mystery and adventure.

I started with sketches, before working on the final books, and we all went back and forth over those. We hit it off right away on the basic ideas, but there were lots of small details to decide on. For instance, I originally had Regie wearing tights over his legs like Superman, and the NKFM said they didn't want that particular detail, so I took off the tights. I showed Regie with

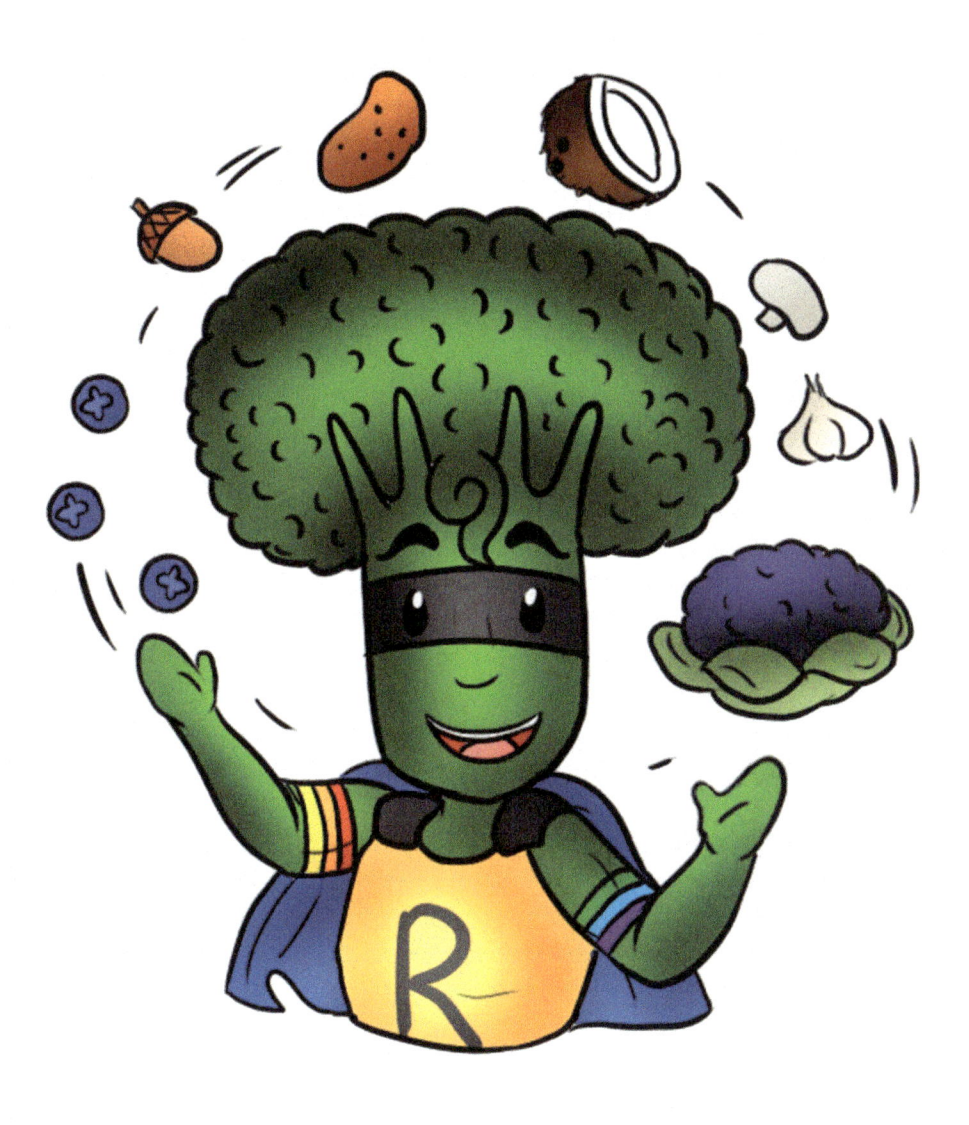

As the National Kidney Foundation of Michigan expands Regie's Rainbow Adventure, the image of the superhero continues to evolve. The illustrations by Emily Zieroth, from late 2016, emphasize Regie's fun and friendly look while maintaining his superhero status—including a Superman-style curl on his forehead.

and without a mask, and we decided we liked him with the mask. Then, as a next step, I completed the Island of Red and submitted that book for approval. The NKFM liked that one, so they asked me to complete the series.

As you read this book, and if you're thinking of working with an illustrator, I do have a few tips to share with you. One is that if you're working with kids, it is worth creating something that's well designed and is bright and colorful, because that really gets kids interested. When you're looking for an illustrator, get a sense of what you want before you pick the person. Look at examples and talk with your team about the basic ideas you're trying to achieve. You wouldn't believe how many times clients contact illustrators without much of a description of what they want—and this can lead to a very long process.

I also recommend working alongside your illustrator as the work progresses. That's how I worked with the National Kidney Foundation of Michigan. Discuss the timeline with your illustrator. Some projects may be very involved, and your illustrator may need a couple of months to finish your project. But, professionals work fairly quickly, and a project like a 10-page book shouldn't take a year. Discuss the timeline so you know what to expect.

I consider my work with Regie to be really a wonderful opportunity with great working relationships. I think one sign of our success is that Regie continues to change in small ways. We're all collaborating on making this superhero the best he can be.

Going on Regie's Adventure

Ken Resnicow, Ph.D., is an Irwin M. Rosenstock collegiate professor of health behavior and health education at the University of Michigan School of Public Health, and a professor of pediatrics in the School of Medicine and president of academic assistance. He also serves as evaluator for the Social Innovation Fund-sponsored portion of Regie's Rainbow Adventure. He wrote the introduction to this book, and here, adds:

I'm enthusiastic about doing the ongoing evaluation of the Regie program because, on a deep level, this program brings together a number of effective strategies for communication and behavior change. The NKFM is in a good position to carry out this program, because it's been a credible, trusted organization in this field for many years. One indication of this is that, as the NKFM team members bring Regie into the classroom, they're not promoting any commercial brands or products. There's a serious topic underlying this work that people respect. Kidney health is very serious, and this important organization is addressing all the related issues in a trusted way—a way that uses lots of fun, creative ideas that kids love.

The team running the Regie program has made a lot of smart choices. Finding Emily Zieroth to illustrate the books was a perfect choice. She really understands the visuals that kids gravitate toward. Her illustrations of Regie communicate the strength and power and also the kindness that is appealing to kids. Then, the NKFM team continues the process of listening and changing as its team members look at the data. Regie himself has been field-tested and the team continues to play with the images and elements of the program and improve them. That's what you need to do with a relatively new program like Regie to make it successful.

Our Story • 35

Crystal D'Agostino, M.S.W., serves as program manager at the National Kidney Foundation of Michigan and oversees all of its early childhood programming, including the Regie's Rainbow Adventure program.

Regie is on the move.

The Regie's Rainbow Adventure program has been in a constant state of growth since it first began. What started as a nutrition and physical education program for children in select counties grew into a program serving thousands of children in multiple counties throughout southeast Michigan.

One of the most important principles that the Regie program was founded on was the desire to truly improve the health and nutrition of children and their families. This intention is at the center of all of the work that we do, and inspires every aspect of our programming. We have found that programming in early childcare centers is especially important because of the remarkable period of growth and development that children within that age range are experiencing. Physical health and nutrition have been identified as important factors in early childhood school development, and nutritional deficiencies impede physical growth and development, thus negatively affecting a child's school readiness. The Early Childhood Standards of Quality document, published by the Michigan State Board of Education, states that the standards for child education must meet the expectations within two learning models: "Approaches to Learning Domain", and "Expectations in Social-Emotional Development." Healthy eating and nutrition education is an Early Learning Expectation. Therefore, the Regie program doesn't just educate children and their families, but it also works to assist early learning providers in providing a complete curriculum.

We recently received a grant to expand the Regie program into Washtenaw County, west of Detroit—and that's just one example of how, and through the years, we've continued building this program. Very carefully, step by step, we build Regie's Rainbow Adventure so that it can be scaled successfully.

Today, we tell teachers and parents: Regie's Rainbow Adventure educates and empowers children, their families and educators to make healthy changes in their childcare centers and homes, so that children are better prepared to enter kindergarten. Through the Social Innovation Fund, in recent years, we're proud that our program has reached those most in need—children and families from schools and neighborhoods that lack healthy food choices, sound nutritional information and other vital health-related resources. Children in these programs learn and adopt nutritional and physical activity behaviors that prevent chronic disease, promote their well-being and, ultimately, place them on a path to join others in a generation of healthy, prepared learners. In working with children aged 3 to 5 and their parents, we have a maximal potential for impact, because the earlier in life we reach people the greater effect the programs can have on their life course.

The stories' main character is the superhero Regie, who we describe as half man and half broccoli. His main superpower is the ability to fly, but he needs to keep building up his own strength so he has the energy to fly to all of the different islands of color. He gets that energy by eating fruits and vegetables and by being physically active. Regie's challenge is to earn all six colored power stripes in the course of his adventures to the six islands. He earns these stripes, which appear on his arms, by eating a fruit or vegetable that corresponds with the color of each island. We provide pictures of Regie with the power stripes, shown in white, so that kids can color in each stripe as they go on the adventures with Regie.

What makes this program truly innovative is that it brings a very high-quality, behaviorally focused, science-based nutrition education into these childhood settings—coupled with rigorous evaluation that continues on a consistent basis. The outcomes we are measuring include changes in nutrition and physical activity related to the child's behavior; the amount of the child's screen time; consumption of sugar-sweetened beverages; and general health indicators.

Past data has shown that the Regie program results in an increase in fruit and vegetable consumption at home, increased physical activity, increased preparation for the next grade, and decreased screen time.

As an organization develops a program as innovative as Regie, many concepts are tested along the way. From fostering relationships with childcare centers to fine-tuning the Regie program to make it as cohesive as it can be, the NKFM staff has worked hard to make the Regie program into the package that it is today. One thing that has made the program so successful has been all of the local childcare directors and providers who have partnered with the NKFM. When Regie first began, it became clear that in order to be successful, we would need to develop strong relationships with local early learning communities. We have been fortunate to have the opportunity to foster partnerships that are mutually enjoyable: We don't just provide the Regie program, but we also work to contribute to any committees and meetings that our partners invite us to. We want our partners to feel supported by us as an organization, not just as a program provider. Our partners have given us the opportunity to carry out our program, and have provided exceptional feedback along the way. It is because of our relationships with them that Regie has been able to grow and improve at all.

The ability to grow and change on a regular basis has been important for the Regie program. Some aspects of the program, tried in the first years of our partnership with the Social Innovation Fund, have now been discontinued. One of those aspects was an effort, in the program's first two years, to provide children and their parents with fruits or vegetables that they could take home each week. We would build on the tasting in the classroom by giving the families the same fruit or vegetable—along with recipes—to try at home. This was popular with parents and, as Regie expands, some communities may want to try this idea again, depending on the resources available to them. Within the design of our Social Innovation Fund partnership, though, we found that that particular outreach to families was not sustainable in our budget. Mainly, it came down to a question of logistics. When we needed that larger quantity of each food delivered to the Head Start centers each week of the Regie series, we found that it was difficult to find produce vendors who could reliably provide that quantity of each fruit and vegetable at an affordable cost. Another element of the planning that became too difficult for us to sustain was how the fruit and vegetables would be handled at each center. Even after we found a vendor to provide that quantity of ripe produce, the fruits and vegetables arrived in bulk and the centers had to figure out how to bag portions, along with our recipes, to send home with the children each week. At smaller sites, this was not so daunting. At a site serving hundreds of children, this became a barrier. While we offered this service, the at-home experience was popular with parents and, as Regie expands, some communities may want to reconsider this option.

Even as we ended the weekly distribution at the Social Innovation Fund-sponsored Regie sites, we continue to offer what we like to call "Regie Paloozas." These began in an effort to increase survey response rates for the evaluation component and to strengthen relationships with center administration employees, teachers and parents. In order to carry out a Regie Palooza, staff members coordinate with center administration and teachers as to when the palooza will take place so that both the front office and classroom teachers are able to direct parents to our table once they have dropped off their child in the classroom. The NKFM staff arrives at the school before children are dropped off. They set up a table with resources, a healthy snack with a corresponding recipe and survey materials. Parents are sometimes wary as they approach, unsure of what it is we actually do and who we are. These Regie Paloozas are a great way to introduce the work the NKFM does and explain the evaluation component of Regie's Rainbow Adventure. Parents are given a gift card and a raffle ticket that enters them into a larger gift card drawing for completing the surveys then and there, before they leave the center. Parents are still eligible to receive the gift card if they return the survey by the due date. The NKFM staff are available to help parents with survey comprehension and any questions they have about the program. Many parents start chatting with staff members about healthy recipes their families enjoy, inquire about other NKFM early childhood programs, or share a fun Regie's Rainbow Adventure-related story about their child. It really is a valuable time to form relationships with parents. These events are held at both pre-program and post-program time points, and have been proven to increase survey response rate as well as the center's satisfaction with NKFM programming.

Throughout all of this work, our team is motivated by trying to help people avoid chronic diseases such as diabetes, high blood pressure and kidney disease. That deep, personal commitment is so important for the people who work here. While growing up, I was always interested in working with people to help make their lives a little better. At first, I thought I might become a teacher. Eventually, I became a social worker and got a job with a large health system, working in the nephrology unit. As a social worker, I helped dialysis patients and their families in high-needs communities. I worked with them in many ways, helping them get their medications or plan transportation back and forth to dialysis. I saw firsthand the huge impact that this problem had on so many lives—both the patients and their families. That's what moved me to volunteer and to raise funds for the National Kidney Foundation of Michigan. Eventually, I was able to work directly for the NKFM. Then, my earlier desire to work with kids became a reality, too. The work I do now is a perfect vocational fit for me. That's why I care so much about seeing the Regie program succeed and grow.

Brandy Gingell is a teacher at the Starfish Family Services Head Start center in Livonia, just west of Detroit. This is her story:

Regie's world invites teachers to go many places with the lessons we develop—far beyond the colored islands in the books. Regie is so exciting for the children that he unlocks countless creative possibilities for us, as teachers. Kids are willing to let Regie take them in many directions.

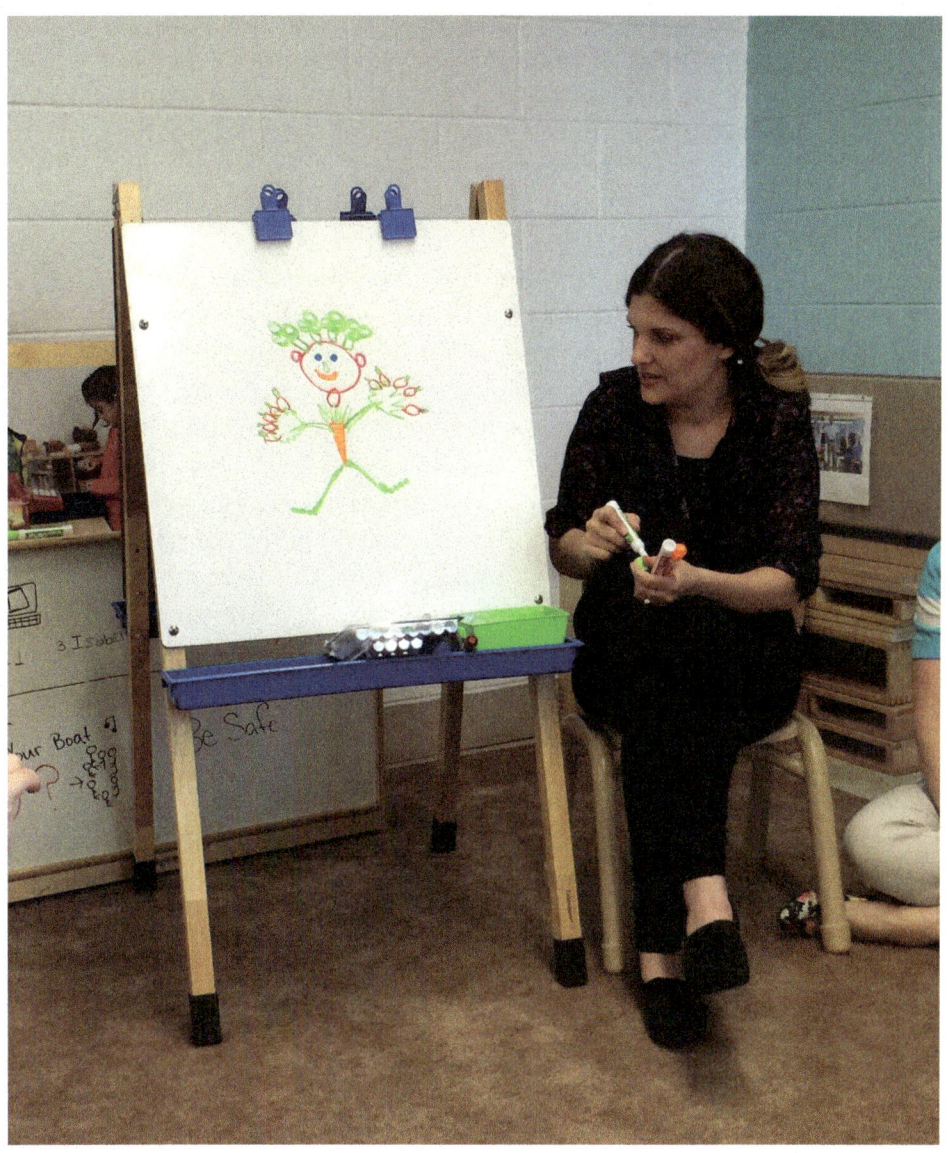

Brandy Gingell sketches on a white board as her Head Start children name different kinds of vegetables that could be combined to create another superhero like Regie. There are many imaginative ways to adapt lessons from the Regie curriculum.

For example, some teachers bring in a single fruit or vegetable to taste during each week of the Regie series. I always try to have three each week, and I try to include both fruits and vegetables in the tasting. Some are a hit every year. Kids love the pineapple! But I always ask them to try some challenging foods, too. I've used fresh mushrooms for the Island of Brown. I've used radishes, which are challenging for some children. And I use fresh papaya, even though I had never even tasted fresh papaya myself until I started doing the Regie series.

I also make a big point of giving the children their power stripes after they've tried a taste of that week's food—and I have the children put them on each other. Teachers handle the power stripes differently, but I cut long strips of colored construction paper and have masking tape handy for the kids. As the kids put on their stripes, they practice working together and they take ownership of the stripes they've earned. They're just strips of paper and masking tape, so they may fall off in the course of moving around the class, but usually I'll see kids trying their best to keep that power stripe on all day. Then, the power stripe is also a great reminder for parents to start a discussion when they pick up their kids at the end of the day. "Oh, I see you've got a green stripe on today! What did you try today?"

There are so many ways Regie can fit into overall lesson plans. I always want to emphasize open-ended questions and encourage children to discuss their diverse responses. I usually give them three foods to taste, so we put up a chart on the wall where each child puts a sticker on the row for his or her favorite food that day. It's not a contest. That's not how the children think about it. This is an opportunity for them to express themselves, which they love to do. So, let's say we've tried a carrot, an orange pepper and cantaloupe in the orange week. I'll go around the circle and ask each child to put a sticker on the row of a favorite food. First, we're showing the kids how to make a chart. Then, we're showing them how to express different tastes. We're also discussing our responses to open-ended questions. Why did you like that one? What was it about this food that you didn't like?

Was it the taste or texture or smell of the food that you liked—or didn't like?

I also invite the children to be a creative part of the process. I might ask the group to help me draw a new kind of vegetable superhero. They'll name fruits and vegetables that could form different parts of this new body. I just did this recently, and we had lettuce leaves for hands and radishes for fingers! We had legs made of green beans and toes made of peas. The kids use their imaginations to take the story further.

One of the most important aspects of the Regie program is the message that children need to keep active to be strong and healthy. We need to help children reduce their level of screen time overall. The evidence now is so clear that time spent in front of the television—and in front of other screens like tablets or video games—has a direct impact on health in childhood. A study published last year by the National Institutes of Health says:

> Excessive TV viewing has been linked to a range of adverse health and behavioral outcomes such as obesity and overweightness, which in turn may cause increased risk of chronic diseases such as cardiovascular disease, diabetes and other metabolic diseases, some cancers, depression and various sleeping difficulties and decreased sleep length. Short-term follow-up studies of students for two to four years suggest negative associations between TV viewing time and measures of school achievement. Furthermore, children who are high TV viewers tend to remain high TV viewers, relative to others, over time, and high level of TV viewing in childhood is associated with health risk factors (e.g., overweightness, poor cardio-respiratory fitness) in adulthood, independent of the adult's levels of TV viewing.[1]

The National Institutes of Health posted a 2015 recommendation that children under age 2 should have no screen time; children over age 2 should be limited to one to two hours of

[1] https://www.ncbi.nlm.nih.gov/pmc/articles/PMC4456860/

screen time appropriate for their age; and that, despite what advertisements may claim, videos aimed at very young children do not help with their development. There are lots of other studies now that draw the same conclusions. Children's excessive screen time is a serious problem. One way to think about this is this way: Children spend so much time with screens now that it amounts to a nearly-full-time job. A Centers for Disease Control and Prevention report says that American children spend an average of more than 4 $\frac{1}{2}$ hours with screens each day, which is more than 30 hours over seven days. More than half of that 4 $\frac{1}{2}$ hours each day is spent staring at a television; the rest of that time is on other kinds of screens.

That's one of the things I like most about Regie: his nonviolence. Kids love superheroes, but a lot of the famous superheroes are involved in violence toward others. Regie stands out as a real contrast to all of that. He's a totally positive superhero.

Even in early childhood, your peers' opinions matter. I can remember this from when I was a child. If my mom was telling me I should like something—or should avoid it—I was always suspicious. I thought: She's my mom. What does she know about the world? Often, we're more influenced—even in early childhood—by other kids. That's why I encourage the kids to express themselves in the classroom about Regie. I know that I've got kids in any class who actually think it's fun to eat "sometimes food." I hear them talking about loving French fries. But I also know that I've usually got a couple of kids who love fruits and vegetables. I have one boy who just loves kale, for example. This gives me an opportunity, as the teacher, to show all the kids that at least some of the kids think fruits and vegetables are fun. The kids who love French fries learn that there are kids who enjoy the taste of vegetables, like kale. They're more likely to try it, too, as a result.

You can see the impact of Regie during lunchtime at our center. Our children wind up eating most of the fruits and vegetables we serve at lunch. This program is very effective if you understand its full potential.

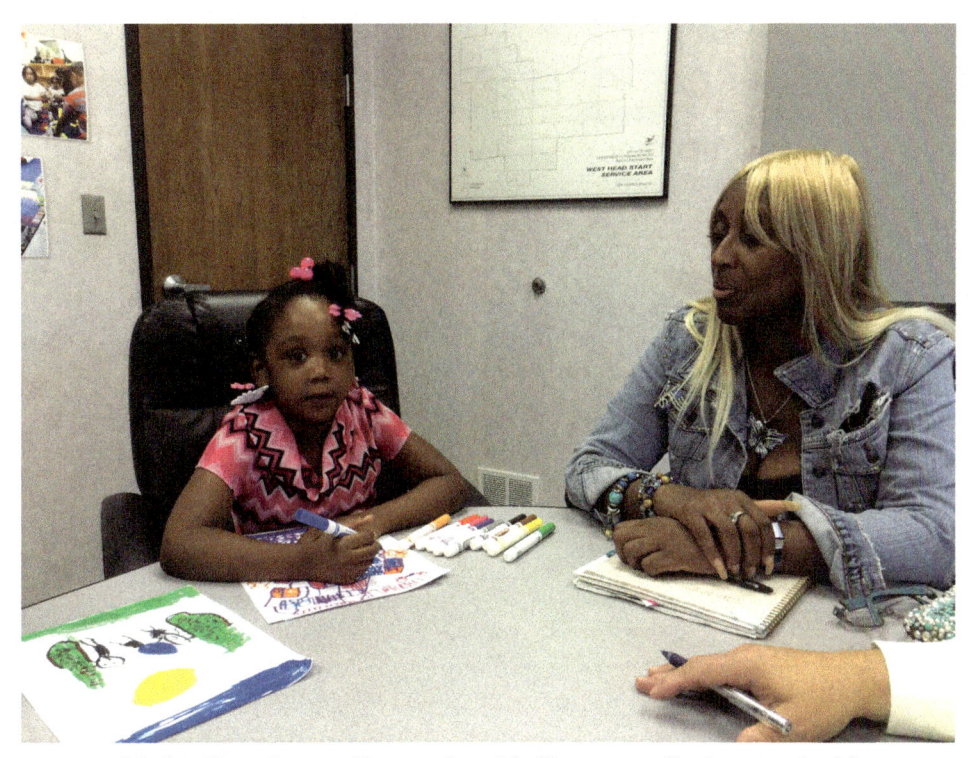

Michai Easterling and her teacher, Ms. Foreman, talk about a colorful floor plan Michai sketched for her dream house—complete with exercise equipment, fresh fruit in the kitchen and room for lots of friends.

Regie's Real Superpower

To bring our story full circle, several of our team members sat down with Debra Foreman, the teacher in the Head Start classroom whom we earlier observed introducing Regie's Island of Purple to her students. We also invited Michai Easterling, from Ms. Foreman's class, along with Michai's mother, Michelle, and Michai's Aunt Monica, who is the nutrition manager at the New St. Paul Tabernacle Head Start Agency. We asked them to talk about the many ways Regie's adventures extend from the classroom into conversations in students' households.

As it turns out, the most eager person in the room is little Michai, who starts the conversation by using colored markers and paper to sketch the floor plan of an ideal home.

"I'm going to show you, right here, my perfect house," she declares, selecting several colors from the box. Because she is sitting next to Ms. Foreman, Michai mainly addresses her description to the teacher, as her small hands sketch spacious walls and then divide the floor plan into many specialized rooms.

"The first thing we want is everybody in the house to love each other—and that means we make room for friends, too. Friends are always welcome in my home," she says, looking up at her teacher. "Ms. Foreman, I'm drawing you here at the front door so you can help welcome people—you know, friends from our class. You can open the door and make sure they're happy. I'm drawing a bell you can ring, if you need to use it. Some of our friends are a little far away. That bell can help call them."

"Oh, I see," Ms. Foreman says. "That bell will be handy. So you want me to welcome people into your home?"

"Yes, and you can show them some of the different rooms. I'm going to make a big playroom for us, but I'm also drawing an exercise room. We need that, too."

"Oh, yes we do. It's good to exercise."

"Exercise makes us strong, so I'm drawing, right here, those big things you lift off the floor to make your arms strong. I've got them in different sizes, here. See? Some of us can lift the big ones; little ones can lift the little ones."

"Oh, yes, I see. You've got weights there—different weights for different people to lift. Oh, yes, that's a good plan."

"Right. And over here, down this hall, is the kitchen, and a big table where we'll eat. Those are red apples on the table, there. Somebody will have to cut them for us. I like my apples cut. And, then, let's go back outside the house." Michai pauses, a marker held in midair, then she nods. "Oh, I've got it! I'll make some swings, too, just outside the house. A set of baby swings for the real little ones and a regular set of swings for us to use. And then, over here, I'm putting apple trees so we can pick more apples anytime we want."

Ms. Foreman nods and offers occasional encouragement as Michai continues the elaborate chart of her ideal home.

"You know," Ms. Foreman says, as she observes Michai's ever-more-complex floor plan, "I grew up here, in Detroit, with fruit trees and gardens. Most people had gardens in their backyards as we were coming up. Then, people forgot about gardens for many years, I think. Now, gardening is coming back in the city—at least in some places. I could take you to some amazing gardens in neighborhoods around Detroit, but the fact is that far too many children are growing up these days without ever seeing a real garden. Kids today think that food is picked from a drive-thru window of a fast-food place. We need more parents to stop and think: What we put into a child's life is what we can expect them to send back out into the world as they grow up. We have to expose children to better foods, because we know what we can expect from a steady diet of fast food and unhealthy snacks, don't we? And it's not good. Part of that lesson for parents is discovering that kids actually do get excited about trying fresh fruits and vegetables—a lot more than parents realize.

"It's true! So many kids are growing up today without any connection to fresh foods." Ms. Foreman motions toward Michai's mother and aunt for support, and they nod in agreement.

"Why, when we were coming up," Ms. Foreman continues, "we all had a garden at home or we knew someone close by in the neighborhood who had a garden. My grandma, Ernestine Pittman, lived right here in Detroit and had a pear tree in her backyard, plus flowers in her garden and this big block of the backyard that was set aside for vegetables. Grandma grew greens, cucumbers, cabbage and tomatoes, and that's where I first learned to love tomatoes and cabbage—and I've loved them all my life because of Grandma. I thank her to this day."

Ms. Foreman pauses, remembering that yard in detail.

"And grapevines, too! I remember she had grapevines down one side of the yard. It was common, back then, for families to have grapes out in the backyard in our neighborhood. And then my mama, Arlesia Foreman, kept that tradition going with her own garden. So many of the foods we ate were right there, growing all around us. I used to love the collards Mama grew and I love the memories I have of watching her bring them in, wash them in the sink, chop them up and put them in a pot for supper. They came out so delicious! And, from other people in the neighborhood, there were other greens. Back then, some grew mustard greens; some grew collards; some grew other vegetables.

"The other big difference was: We ate our meals around a table. Now you go into homes and you'll see people eating all over the place. Often, you might see the child eating near the TV—and maybe Mom is eating something in the kitchen. Growing up, it was so important for us to break bread together. That was absolutely the way we thought of eating—fresh foods, nutritious foods, eating together. Coming up, I don't even recall eating fast food like kids do today."

"Regie provides a powerful opportunity for parents to talk about food with children," says Michai's mother. "I still remember the first time Michai came up to me and started talking about this Regie superhero. At first, I thought it was some cartoon on a TV show she had seen. But Michai said, 'No, Regie's at school.' So, I asked my sister, Monica, about this. I told her, 'Whoever this Regie is—Michai is sure excited about him.' And Monica explained the whole program.

"Week after week, Michai would come home all excited to tell me things about food—like I didn't know anything about fruits and vegetables. It was fun! This was all new to her and she just assumed I didn't know anything about the importance of eating these foods. We enjoyed our talks about Regie. She took it seriously. Michai was the one who told me she wanted to try broccoli, and to this day she loves broccoli. It's so common for parents to have their kids insist on eating their favorite foods and refuse to eat other foods. If you let that happen, you can get down to some very limited tastes. That's what I liked best about Regie: Michai came to *me* and wanted to talk about trying new foods. We did that—at her request—and she loved it. I learned that she likes some vegetables I never would have expected her to like. It's healthy for all of us."

Michai's Aunt Monica is the nutrition manager for the New St. Paul Agency and works closely with the NKFM and the Head Start teachers on the Regie program each year. She has had the opportunity to see Regie implemented, and understands the great impact that Regie has on child development. In Michigan, the Board of Education sets standards for children and expects that they will meet these standards. For children in the early childhood setting, they are expected to learn about nutrition and begin to develop behaviors that contribute to good health. Regie helps kids meet these standards through the encouragement of fruit and vegetable consumption, and also through physical activity. However, the program also helps children learn their colors as Regie travels to different islands, and helps them develop their counting and recall skills. The book encourages kids to count together, and teachers often ask follow-up questions that challenge children to remember the events in the story. These are all skills that children need to practice and develop as they continue to grow.

Monica also reports that the program is so enjoyable because it is easy for teachers to implement. The books are exciting and brief, and are easy to incorporate into the day. If teachers have questions or issues, they can always refer to the manual, or contact NKFM staff. She does believe that it's important to work closely with other staff members, as conducting the Regie program can take some planning.

"I would tell anyone interested in this that they should work cooperatively with others on the planning for the seven weeks of the Regie curriculum," she says. "On the administrative end, you need to think creatively about the fruits and vegetables you can get to go along with the program. You want to find fruits and vegetables children don't already know—but you have to make sure you can get these in your area in the season the teachers are doing the Regie program. Sometimes Regie sessions may come in the winter; sometimes Regie comes in the spring. At the same time, we're thinking about the students who probably are going to experience Regie more than one year in their time with Head Start, so we want to keep bringing them new foods."

Monica continues, "I really like the way the NKFM encourages us all to work together in making these choices. I would say one of our biggest hits was the kiwi—just to give you an example of a fruit that worked out very well."

Ms. Foreman smiles and nods.

"The kiwi was a real surprise for the children!" she says. "You know, it comes with this brown fuzzy skin and the children make all kinds of predictions about what we'll find when we cut it open. They just can't believe it when we show them it's bright green and has these little black seeds."

"I love kiwi, now!" chimes in Michai. "I thought it was going to be brown inside—but it's not."

"Pineapple has been another big hit!" says Monica.

"Pineapple was very interesting!" Ms. Foreman agrees. "Most children only know pineapple in the form that comes out of a can. We started with a whole pineapple that day and the kids were so surprised when we cut that open! We got a really good, ripe, sweet pineapple so, when we cut it up into samples, they did finally recognize the taste. It was a big surprise to connect the taste they already knew with that great, big pineapple we started with on our table."

"We've also made a few choices that didn't go over so well," says Monica. "I remember snap peas weren't a hit. We tried star fruit one time, because they look so unusual, you know—like a star, when you cut them into slices. But the children didn't enjoy them. And, if you're considering trying this program, you also should remember that the Regie program focuses on trying fruits and vegetables in their fresh state. One time, we made a mistake by bringing in eggplant for the Island of Purple. We tried to quickly cook pieces of eggplant before we let the kids sample it, and that didn't work out very well—the kids didn't care for it. So, no more eggplant for us! Mainly, though, the kids love what we bring them. The main thing is to keep talking to the teachers and hear what works best. It's a cooperative effort."

Ms. Foreman adds, "It's also important for the teachers to encourage the children." She turns to Michai and says, "What do we always say in class, if someone doesn't want to take a taste? What do we say?"

"We say, 'You can always take a no-thank-you bite!'" Michai says.

"And what is that?" Ms. Foreman asks.

"Well, you have to try the food, like Ms. Foreman says, and you always know that if you really don't like it, then you can say, 'No thank you,' before eating any more." Then, Michai looks up at Ms. Foreman knowingly, and adds, "But it doesn't work that way, does it? What happens mostly is the bite tastes good."

"And if the first bite doesn't taste good, what else do we say?"

"We say, 'Take two bites.' Because we know the first bite may not be that good. But if you take that second bite—that's when you might really like it!" Michai explains. "It's like when we had to try tomatoes. I took a no-thank-you bite—and that time I just didn't like it. I didn't like all those seeds in that tomato—and I didn't like the skin on the tomato. Then, Ms. Foreman told me to take two bites—and, after the second bite, I discovered I really liked the taste of the tomato's juice, as I chewed it up. That's how it works. Mostly, you wind up liking it."

Ms. Foreman puts an arm around Michai and smiles broadly at her student.

"Michai, what would you say you like best about Regie?" she asks.

"Well," says Michai, "the fact is, he's a superhero. So, you've got to like that. He travels so far and has so many friends! I like his green hair. And I like that he's friendly to everyone—even those friends who are all different types of fruits and vegetables. He likes them all."

Ms. Foreman says, "That's a good way of putting it, Michai. Regie brings a whole lot of components together. Children love superheroes; they love colors. At this age, children want to use all of their senses that are developing so powerfully—and Regie lets them use all of their senses in one experience. Then there's the travel. The children we work with don't get to travel, but Regie gives us this awesome invitation to imagine all kinds of travel. Plus, the big message is: When you travel, you'll find unusual people who will welcome you to their different lands. These are not just stories to these children. This is a big adventure they're excited to take with Regie.

"Anytime you can relate an educational program to children's main interests, it's a powerful opportunity for learning. Think about the most popular video games today for kids of this age—they're all colorful adventure games. Kids love this idea—so much so that they just can't wait to get home and tell Mom or Auntie or Grandma all about the big adventures with Regie. We equip the children with many tangible reminders, as well. We give them stickers. They love stickers! We make little passports that they fill with colorful stickers of fruits and vegetables they've tried. We teach them a song to sing. We show them counting with fruits and vegetables. We show them how Regie moves. Regie really represents this large scaffolding on which we are able to place so many elements that allow children and their parents to connect with these new interests and ideas.

"As teachers, that's our mission. We are entrusted with educating young minds. We do that through the lessons we cover in class, but we also are trying to convey to the adults at home—to Mom and Dad and Grandma and Auntie—that they play a powerful role in their children's growth and learning, as well. They are their child's first teachers. What's great about Regie is that the kids get so excited about him that they actually become teachers themselves. Look at the things Michai has learned and carried back home with her. It's clear that she's going to continue telling Regie's story to everyone she meets. She's going to talk about the need to eat your fruits and vegetables to feel good inside. Those of us who are older and can remember growing up with gardens in our families—we can remember the parents and grandparents who taught us about eating good foods. Michai and her mom are doing that together now. And, I can tell you: That's something that will go on for the rest of Michai's life.

Maria Houroian, M.S.W., serves as a program coordinator for early childhood programs at the National Kidney Foundation of Michigan and is the program lead for Regie's Rainbow Adventure. This is her story:

Have you figured out Regie's real superpower?

Regie has the power to get entire families talking about nutrition. Everyone who meets Regie smiles and enjoys the fun ideas he represents. We naturally want to talk about him and his adventures with the people around us. Before we know it, we're actually talking about nutrition with our families and friends.

There's one notion that our team members at the National Kidney Foundation of Michigan all share: This is more than a job to us. Like Crystal D'Agostino, I'm a social worker, because all my life I've wanted to help people. Yes, Regie is a complex program that combines the best educational strategies with rigorous evaluation. But, to put it simply: We've fallen in love with Regie. It's a sign of how effective he is.

I work on the front lines with Regie. In our agency, the title "program lead" means that I'm designated to work directly with Regie sites. I assist in grant writing, filing reports, scheduling, training and all other aspects of the program. Then, if people at my sites have questions along the way, I'm the one they contact.

Ninety percent of the time we hear positive things from the teachers. Overall, they're thrilled with the program. Sometimes they do have questions or concerns—in the past, the main concerns have been about getting produce deliveries organized in an effective way each week. I also handle requests for personal appearances of Regie. Our sites have the opportunity to ask Regie to come visit at some point throughout the year. We offer this as a parent engagement opportunity for the centers. If a center is hosting a game night or a reading event, or another event where they'd like the superhero to attend and engage with the children, centers can ask someone to dress up as the superhero. The NKFM provides the costume, as well as some information for the person who is playing Regie. Then, the individual dresses up as Regie and talks to the kids about fruits and vegetables, as well as being active. Some sites want Regie to visit every year; other sites run the program without an appearance. If I get a request for an appearance, then I work with the staff at the site. I ask, "Do you have a parent or a teacher who would be interested in appearing as Regie?" Most of the time, staff members select a parent to play the role. Even if that parent is hesitant at first—I've talked with a lot of them afterward—they have a blast being a superhero. We have a total of a half-dozen costumes, and we'd like to have more made as we expand. Right now, a site needs to give us about a month's notice for us to coordinate the costume with the volunteer playing Regie.

Working with this superhero just makes you want to talk with family and friends about the foods we eat. I've often thought back to my nona's garden and the fun of picking and cooking vegetables from her backyard. It's still a great idea to think about planting a garden, if that is possible where you live. It can help you eat healthier and on a budget. This whole idea comes naturally to me, since I grew up enjoying sports and eating healthy foods—sometimes right out of the garden.

What we're teaching children today are the lessons I was taught by my nona—my grandmother who came from Italy when she was young. My parents didn't have a garden at our house, but Nona did, and she often babysat us when we were little, so that was part of my life growing up. Grandpa always planted the huge garden every year and Nona was in charge of picking what we were going to eat and then cooking it up for dinner. I remember walking through the garden amongst cucumbers and tomatoes and different types of herbs. Nona set aside part of their basement for a big cupboard that she filled, each year, with jars of homemade tomato sauce. She cooked many different things, including pasta and chicken cacciatore—but, surprisingly, her greens were my all-time favorite. Even as a preschooler, I loved how she made them. It wasn't fancy, but it was so good. When I was little, I loved the taste of the browned garlic in the greens—and the way the long pieces of cooked greens would twirl on my fork. I even had an opportunity, recently, to go back to Nona's house and spend time talking with her about making those greens. She had never written down a recipe. Why would she have? She knew it by heart. I had fun, as an adult, watching her make greens and actually helping her record the recipe.

Finally, I have to say: When we were little, Nona didn't just entice us with food. She was very assertive. You always had to at least taste everything on your plate before you could leave the table. That's an idea she instilled in me as a preschooler and it's the kind of value we're teaching today, through Regie. So, here is Nona's recipe for greens. You know what to do: Go on, take a taste! It's healthy for you!

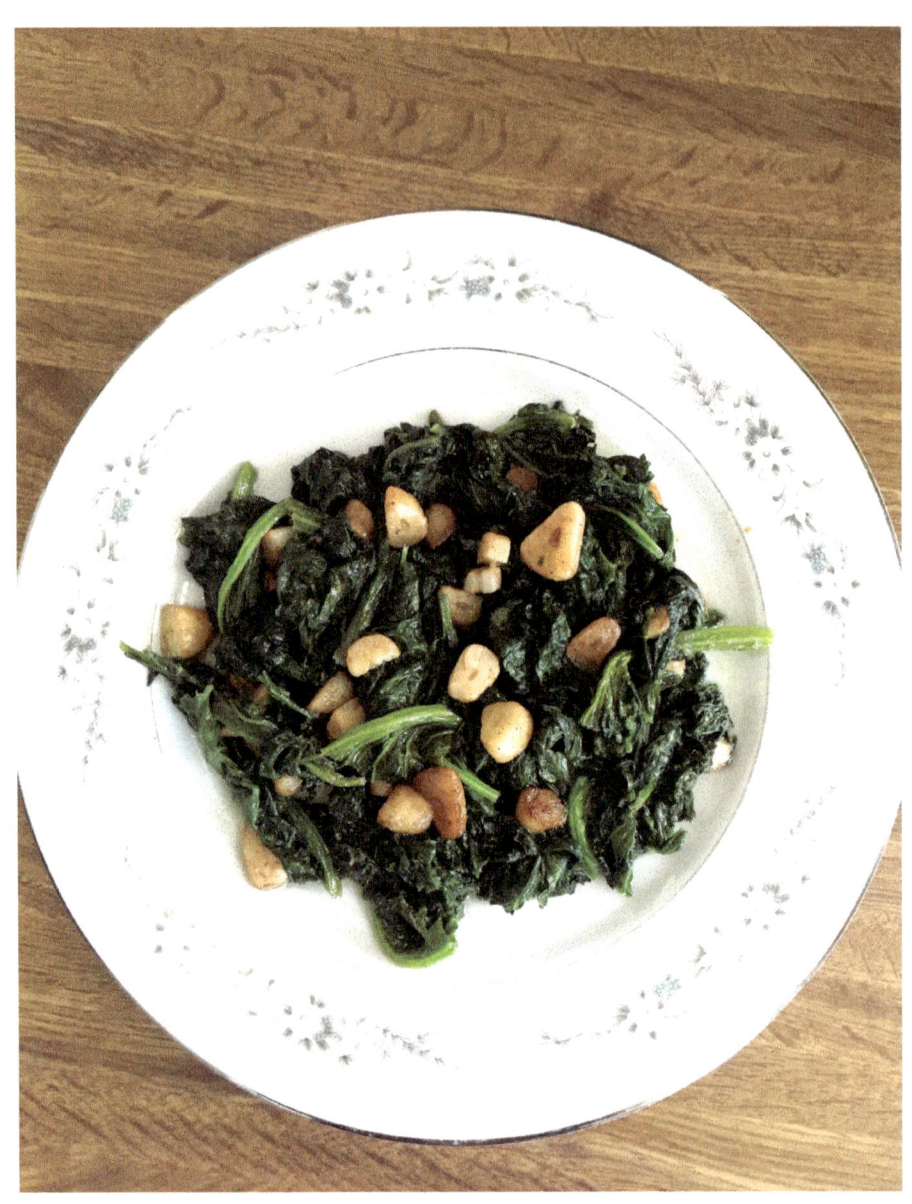

Nona's greens.

Nona's Greens

- 1 bunch mustard or collard greens, washed, with hard stems torn off
- 1 bulb garlic (approximately 12 to 14 cloves)
- ¾ cup water
- Olive oil sufficient to coat the bottom of the pan
- Salt and pepper, to taste

Chop the greens.

Cut each garlic clove into 2 or 3 pieces.

Coat the bottom of a large pan with olive oil.

Sauté the garlic until golden brown.

Add the greens to the pan. Heat and stir until the greens wilt. Add salt and pepper to taste.

Add the water and bring to a boil over medium heat. Cover the pan and cook for about 10 minutes.

Add more water if needed.

It's a Bird! It's a Plane! It's Regie!

Want to see Regie in action? Want to get friends and neighbors excited about bringing this program to your community?

To accompany this book, we produced a four-minute introductory video, which is easy to share via YouTube. In this video, you'll see:

- A typical Regie appearance, portrayed by a parent at one of our Detroit sites
- Monica Easterling talking about the challenge of introducing a healthy approach to nutrition to preschool children and their families
- Parent and site manager Monique Snyder describing the responses of children
- Gabrielle Johnson a teacher and parent, explaining the multi-faceted value of Regie—including early literacy through the book series
- Chief science officer, Dr. Arthur Franke, talking about underlying health issues and then later summarizing the National Kidney Foundation of Michigan's plan to expand the Regie program

You can contact us anytime through http://www.nkfm.org/

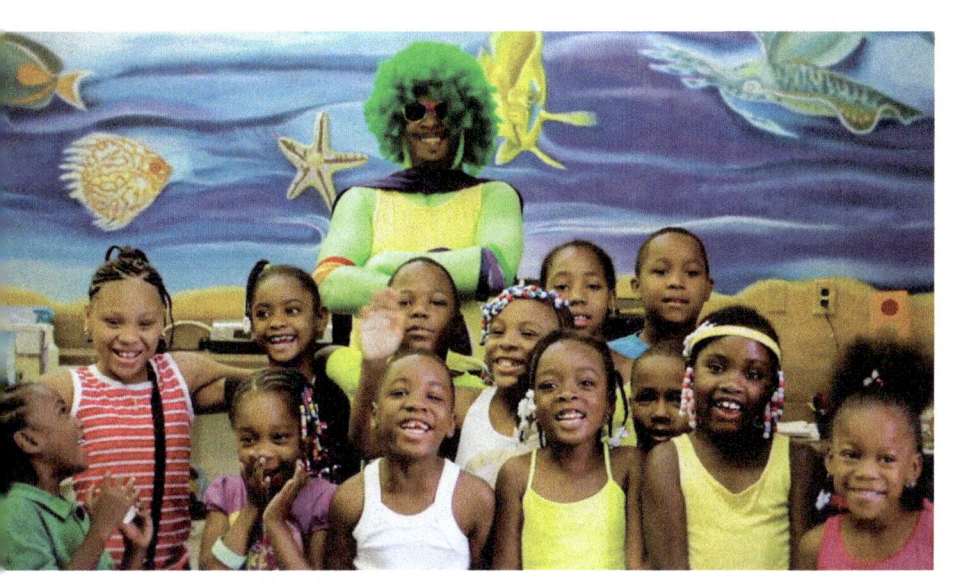

A scene from the new National Kidney Foundation of Michigan video about Regie's Rainbow Adventure.
Watch: youtube.com/watch?v=SJmxnVL5Ew4&

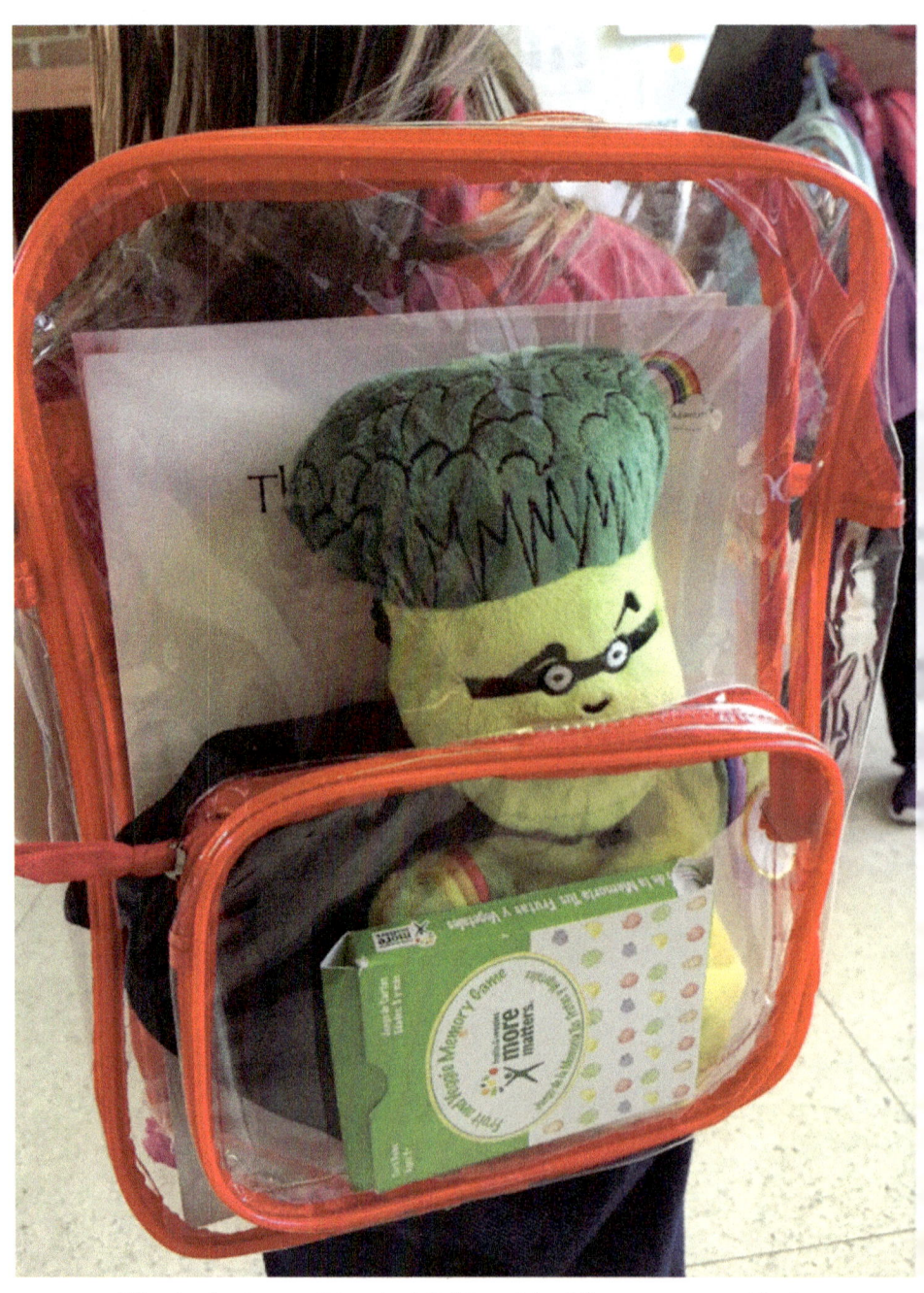

The site leader at a Livonia, Michigan Head Start came up with the creative idea to make a Regie backpack for families to sign out and take home. This allows the children the ability to share their Regie experiences with their families outside of the classroom.

Our Resources

The books in this series, sponsored through the Corporation for National and Community Service's Social Innovation Fund, include examples of resources developed by our organizations so that we may provide you with a clearer sense of our work.

From Maria Houroian, M.S.W., who serves as a program coordinator for early childhood programs at the National Kidney Foundation of Michigan and is the program lead for Regie's Rainbow Adventure®:

The ongoing quality of Regie's Rainbow Adventure depends on the materials and training we provide to the sites we serve. We now have eight people who are able to conduct Regie training across the region that we serve, as each year, site leaders contact us to schedule this training for their teachers and their teaching assistants. A full training session takes approximately one hour, and we most often administer a full session at sites with new staff members, because we want everyone to completely understand the program. For a full training, we bring a laptop and projector and we take the staff through all the background of the Regie program and all of its components. Teachers who are new to the program need to understand why we're doing this, so we cover topics like the increase in childhood obesity and its causes. If we're going to a site where Regie has been running for a while, we might decide to present a refresher session of about 30 minutes. In this quicker version of training, we're focused on bringing fresh materials, reviewing all current available options and discussing any updates that were made since the previous year. Because this program is so much fun—not to mention effective and successful—we're making many return visits now. As we expand, we know we'll also have more new sites to serve with the complete training sessions.

Most of the classrooms we serve have two teachers: usually, a lead teacher and an assistant. Each classroom team gets one new bag of materials each year.

Want to Become Regie?

Centers that participate in the Regie Rainbow Adventure program have access to a costume that they can rent for special appearances. This interaction with a "real life Regie" provides children with an additional opportunity to talk about being healthy. Below is information provided to center volunteers or parents who agree to dress up as Regie.

Thank you for agreeing to dress up as Regie Rainbow today!

It is great that you are interested in talking to kids about being healthy, eating fruits and vegetables, and the importance of physical activity. Children enjoy meeting Regie, the superhero broccoli, and hearing about his adventures. Please use any of the ideas listed below as talking points when interacting with children today. You don't need to read from this page—just have a lot of energy! We are so excited for you to move and groove as Regie Rainbow! Thank you!

Regie Rainbow travels to different islands on an adventure. At the first six islands, he eats fruits and vegetables to give him energy. He also performs physical activities throughout his adventure. In the seventh book, he learns that it is important to watch less TV and be more physically active. Regie enjoys healthy foods and moving his body. This program also focuses on the colors of the rainbow, counting and using manners. Feel free to incorporate any of these topics when acting as Regie.

Talking points for Regie

These discussion starters can be used with individual children or in a group setting. Feel free to adapt these ideas so they are appropriate to the children's most recent week with Regie:

- "I had a banana this morning. What did you eat this morning?"
- "What did you learn about fruits and vegetables from reading my adventures?"

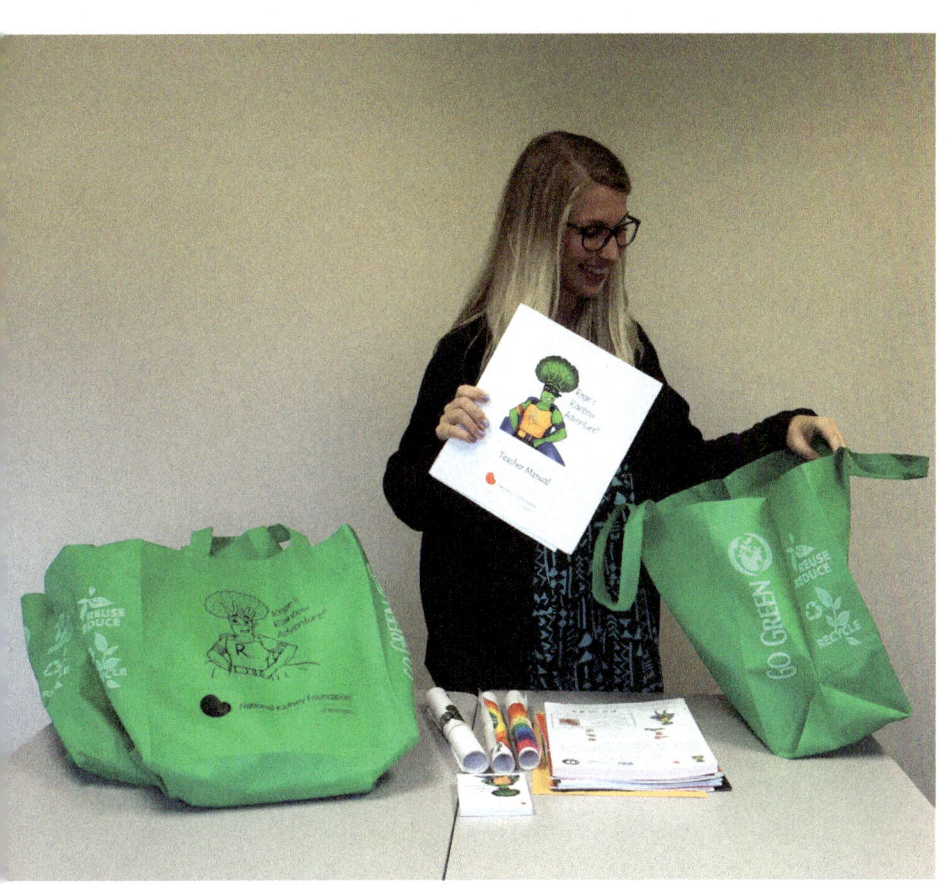

Each year, the National Kidney Foundation of Michigan staff pack bags with all the materials teachers need to present Regie's Rainbow Adventure, including a teacher's manual, colorful storybooks, posters and introductory handouts for parents.

- "What is your favorite red vegetable?"
- "Have you ever tried a kiwi? Did you like it?"
- "I can jump up and down 10 times. How many times can you jump up and down?"
- "What physical activities do you like to do?"
- "Have you helped your mom or dad make dinner before? Tell me what you did."

Our Resources • 63

Optional physical activities

Here are some ideas to get children up and moving with you:
- Play a game of "Regie Says" (just like "Simon Says").
- Play "Red Light/Green Light."
- Dance to music.
- Move like animals (leap like a frog, hop like a kangaroo, etc.).
- Have a balance competition by lifting one foot off the ground.
- Sing and move to "Head, Shoulders, Knees, and Toes."
- Have children do the chicken dance, the Macarena or the hokey pokey.
- Have children practice counting while doing any of these movements: jumping jacks, hopping, marching in place, jumping rope, shimmying, swimming, being an airplane, riding bikes in place, dancing, making arm circles, tapping their shoulders, doing shoulder rolls, touching their knees and toes, clapping their hands and tapping their sides.
- Use your imagination or ask the children to suggest movements they enjoy.

More things you can do

- Talk about the benefits of eating healthy foods and being physically active. You don't have to go into much detail; basic information is fine.
- Look at the teacher's manual for the program for additional ideas and talking points.
- Role model healthy behaviors, like trying a new food, eating fruits and vegetables and being physically active.
- Discuss Regie's friends, his adventure and what he learned from his experience.

Eating the colors of the rainbow

From Maria Houroian

Children absolutely love our "Eating the colors of the rainbow" song. They sing it even after the Regie series ends. As we visit sites for training, I have even heard children singing the song while they are lining up in a hallway. It's wonderful to hear our song take on such a life of its own because the kids love it. Sing to the tune of "Twinkle, Twinkle Little Star." Here is are the lyrics:

> Red, orange, yellow, green and blue
>
> Shiny purple, too.
>
> All the colors that we know
>
> Living inside the rainbow.
>
> Red, orange, yellow, green and blue
>
> Shiny purple, too.

Recommended Websites

When teachers and parents ask for more information, our Regie team recommends these respected websites:
- https://www.nkfm.org/regierainbow
- https://www.facebook.com/Regie.Rainbow
- http://www.letsmove.gov/
- https://healthykidshealthyfuture.org/
- https://www.choosemyplate.gov/

Warm Sweet Potato and Apple Bake

- 3 cups washed and sliced sweet potatoes
- 3 cups washed and sliced apples (about 2 large)
- 1 tablespoon brown sugar
- juice of 1 lemon
- ¾ teaspoon ground cinnamon
- ¼ teaspoon ground cloves, allspice or nutmeg
- ¼ teaspoon salt
- dash of pepper
- 1 tablespoon melted butter

Heat oven to 400 F.

In a medium-size bowl, mix together sweet potatoes and apples.

In a separate small bowl, squeeze lemon for juice and mix in melted butter, brown sugar, salt, and spices.

Pour lemon juice, butter and spices over apple and potato mixture and mix everything together.

Place all ingredients into medium-size baking dish and cover with foil.

Bake for 45 minutes, or until potatoes and apples are soft when poked with a fork. (**Tip**: Halfway through baking (about 20 minutes), carefully take the pan out and use a spoon to pour any juices back onto the mixture, then return the dish to the oven.)

Carrot Cake Oatmeal Cookies

- 1 cup instant oats
- ¾ cup whole-wheat flour
- 1 ½ teaspoons baking powder
- 1 tablespoon ground cinnamon
- ⅛ teaspoon salt
- 2 tablespoons canola or vegetable oil
- 1 large egg
- 1 teaspoon vanilla extract
- ½ cup sugar
- 1 cup grated carrots
- ½ cup crushed pineapple
- ½ cup raisins (optional)

Heat oven to 325 F. Grease or line a baking sheet with parchment paper.

In a medium-size bowl, combine the oats, flour, baking powder, cinnamon, and salt.

In a separate bowl, whisk together the oil, egg, vanilla and sugar. Mix in the pineapple.

Combine the flour mixture with the egg mixture. Fold in the carrots and raisins.

Chill the dough for at least 30 minutes. If longer, cover with plastic wrap

Drop teaspoons of the dough into the prepared cookie sheet.

Bake for 12-15 minutes. Cool on the baking sheet for at least 15 minutes.

Store in an airtight container for up to one week.

Our Partners

Why this matters so much to us

From Dr. Herman B. Gray, M.D., MBA, President and CEO of United Way for Southeastern Michigan:

As the father of two thriving adult children, I fully understand the challenges of parenting. Even under the best of circumstances, parenting is the most difficult, and yet fulfilling, duty that many of us will face.

My wife, Shirley, and I had it pretty easy with our two girls, but of course, there were always challenges. Homework time was a battleground as the girls struggled with math. These were moments that tested me. (They also proved that I would've made a terribly impatient tutor.) And like many parents, we dealt with stubbornness from our youngest, who pronounced "I know that" to everything that came her way, whether she truly did or not.

I wasn't alone in these moments. As a pediatrician, I saw that the parents of my young patients shared the same worries as me, and I sympathized with them. They would often ask questions like:

"Will they get into the 'right' school?"

"Will they be happy?"

"Will they make a good living?"

My role was to offer nonjudgmental support, accurate advice and reassurance. Perhaps one of the greatest parenting challenges is helping our children develop good judgment, moral character and intellectual strength.

It is a tough business raising a child.

Whether a child is 6 or 60, parenting never truly ends, but I am proud to say that both of my girls graduated from the University of Michigan—one earning a master's degree and another a law degree. It makes me proud to see my children passionately pursuing and leading in their careers.

Every child deserves the opportunity to succeed, and it is our collective responsibility to support them. That is why our Social Innovation Fund work is so important. It's structured to create best-in-class practices to help parents and caregivers access the resources and tools needed to support the children in their lives. This work has the potential to not only affect our local community, but it can influence nationwide policy as well.

If we do not move forward to meet the challenges of our ever-changing world, we will fall behind. We cannot be afraid to try new or different approaches to age-old social conditions. Our community's success depends on how we care for and develop our children, which is why it is crucial that we work together and use creative strategies to prepare them for a global future.

My work at United Way for Southeastern Michigan (UWSEM) means a great deal to me. I am fully committed to the service of others and to making the world our children live in a better place. We can only carry out this work with our dedicated partners and with the support of our community, and I am grateful for the opportunity we have to collaborate with and learn from one another.

At United Way, we embrace our legacy as leaders in social innovation, and we move forward confidently into an unknown future, growing and learning, and always serving. I hope the books in *The Bib to Backpack Learning Series* will help to guide many parents and community leaders in how we might achieve our goals together – and create a brighter future for our children.

Herman Gray, M.D., MBA, is president and CEO of United Way for Southeastern Michigan, appointed to his current post in 2015. Before that, he served as the executive vice president of pediatric health services at the Detroit Medical Center (DMC); prior, he was the DMC Children's Hospital of Michigan's president and chief executive officer for eight years, after serving as its chief operating officer and chief of staff. Dr. Gray's areas of specialty include health care administration, public health,

child advocacy and nonprofit management. His medical degree was from the University of Michigan and his Master of Business Administration was from the University of Tennessee. He and his wife, Shirley, have two daughters.

> **Tip for Success: Five Themes to Stress With Your Potential Supporters**
>
> Most nonprofits face the twin challenges of raising funds and recruiting participants. Consider including these themes as you reach out:
>
> 1. Innovation — How does your team transform and adapt ideas as you encounter inevitable challenges?
> 2. Evidence — How do you know your program works? How is your program designed to shift gears on the basis of new evidence?
> 3. Scale — How can your program expand? How do you expect to flexibly adapt to the challenges you face as you grow?
> 4. Match — How can you add additional or matching dollars and why will those new funders choose to join your effort?
> 5. Knowledge Sharing — How are you contributing to the widespread sharing of fresh ideas and best practices?
>
> *Adapted from the SIF Communicators Toolkit*

Tips from United Way and the Social Innovation Fund

In 2009, the Social Innovation Fund (SIF) was launched through the Corporation for National and Community Service (CNCS), the federal agency that sponsors many service programs, including AmeriCorps, Learn and Serve America and Senior Corps. What made CNCS's new SIF initiative distinctive in the existing array of federal programs was three of its core goals: a commitment to collaborate with already existing nonprofits across the country, rather than creating new federal programs from scratch; a strong mandate to include ongoing collection of data and evaluation of each funded program to demonstrate effectiveness; and a pledge to widely share information that could foster scaling and replication of similarly effective programs. The book you are reading is a major part of United Way for Southeastern Michigan's effort to reach that third goal. The six books in what we are calling *The Bib to Backpack Learning Series* provide transparent and detailed information on how the programs of our six Metro Detroit partners began, how they overcame challenges along the way and how the programs are structured today. The books themselves are easily accessible doorways into our programs — and into the larger potential of the SIF. In addition, by producing high-quality books that share the story of the programs, we also are equipping our six regional nonprofit partners with a valuable tool for their ongoing work with community leaders and funders. Each of these nonprofit groups now can say that they literally are "writing the book" on how to help with early education in challenging neighborhoods through ongoing innovation. That's a major boost in convincing additional partners to support this work.

If you are thinking about developing a program in your region, you also will want to explore the hundreds of pages of tips and detailed analysis of existing programs that are shared by the SIF at http://www.nationalservice.gov/programs/social-innovation-fund/knowledge-initiative/reports. These online SIF materials are free to download in PDF format and are packed with helpful information about strategies that already are working in communities from coast to coast. Since one goal of this fund is to encourage robust sharing of information, you may even discover programs in your region that could collaborate with your group in the future.

If you explore the federal website, you will find details on two programs with similar-sounding names that are administered by CNCS. The original 2009 SIF, which is supporting the six programs in southeast Michigan, is sometimes referred to as "SIF Classic" to distinguish it from a new program that was launched in 2014 that is called "SIF Pay for Success." That newer program changes the funding model to leverage federal money only after other organizations have established a program and have proven that it works. The Detroit-area programs are part of the original SIF — but, at this point, either fund may interest community leaders in your part of the country. Both are covered on the federal website.

The following helpful ideas are paraphrased from several public reports, including a late-2015 analysis called *State of the SIF Report*, the *SIF Communicators Toolkit* and a *Lessons and Stories* report, focused on United Way.

> Question: Has your involvement with the SIF, including the evaluation component, helped you when meeting with funders?
>
> Answer from UWSEM: Education and youth development is a major focus in our region, and funders also understand the value of SIF. The quality of the SIF's mandated evaluations are especially appealing to many funders who are now expecting to see increased levels of accountability tied to their funds. The national prominence of the SIF, coupled with the fact that this connects with a major focus in our region, has allowed our fund development teams to feel comfortable approaching both funders we work with consistently as well as establishing new relationships with groups that want to contribute to the well-being of children and families in our region.
>
> Question: How has your involvement with the SIF enabled your organization to scale your programs?
>
> Answer from UWSEM: We are continuing to work on scaling efforts with our six programs, including the program that is the subject of this book: Regie's Rainbow Adventure. We work with our six organizations in a collaborative way to set scaling and replication goals and to design action plans to reach those goals. We provide each organization with additional staff hours and technical assistance. In 2016, our major effort toward this goal is the creation of this series of six

books that will help community leaders nationwide understand how they could replicate these programs. We are also committed to spreading the use of the valuable Ages and Stages Questionnaire through our BibToBackpack.org website. Plus, we continue to gather new data that help us to identify additional communities in need of these early childhood interventions. That will guide the future placement of resources from our current programs.

Question: When telling the story of an organization's current work and its goals in the future, who should be addressed on a regular basis?

Answer from the SIF: Most organizations maintain a list of "target audiences" as they communicate about their work. Take a look at your list to see if it includes:

- Board members – These leaders set the overall direction of your organization and secure ongoing funding. Members of your board need to understand your work and need to know key details they can share as ambassadors for your program.
- Private funders – Your relationship with your funders doesn't end when the money is provided. These funders are gateways to future funding and they need to know that their money is supporting effective, ongoing work.
- Elected officials – These community leaders can help you overcome barriers and, at some levels of government, may be able to appropriate future funding. Consider scheduling a reception or special program to give elected officials an opportunity to understand your work.
- Program beneficiaries and stakeholders – These men and women embody your impact in the community, but they may not understand the full scope of what you are accomplishing if you don't tell them. Also, help them to understand their ongoing role in telling your group's story.
- Social sector influencers – Are you regularly reaching out to academic institutions, other nonprofit organizations,

for-profit social enterprises and other thought leaders in your community? Do you know local journalists and media personalities with an interest in your core community? Many groups overlook valuable contacts with these influential individuals and institutions, partly because you may not be updating and expanding your list of contacts on a regular basis.

> **Four Tips for Communicating With Your Community**
>
> 1. Communicate regularly – Many organizations are so busy running their programs that they forget there is a larger community that wants to support what they are doing. Consider updates through social media, a monthly newsletter or some other form of ongoing communication.
> 2. Focus on real people – The strongest public response to your work will come when people see the difference your program makes in the lives of the men, women and children involved. This book is an example of offering human stories as a doorway through which people can explore what you are doing.
> 3. Share information – Expand the boundaries of your "external communication" to include opportunities for your team to meet with teams from other similar groups. Share innovations and insights.
> 4. Get creative – Many lengthy reports are generated in a huge program like the SIF. These are essential to track and analyze our evidence, but we also need to find creative, compelling formats for sharing our stories. This series of books is an experiment in sharing of our stories with the world.
>
> *Adapted from the SIF Communicators Toolkit*

Why United Way is an effective partner

Wherever you are in the world, as you read this book, consider inquiring about the international network of United Way affiliates as a starting point in your efforts to launch a program.

For almost 130 years, United Way affiliates have been leaders in charitable giving focused on meeting pressing community needs in the United States and beyond. Tracing its founding to 1887 in Denver, Colorado, these emerging regional programs bore many names, including Community Chest, a phrase familiar to fans of the classic board game, Monopoly.

A major center in the history of United Way innovation was Detroit, following World War II. That's when financial expert Walter C. Laidlaw adapted lessons from his work with World War II war chest drives to begin building a wide-reaching community consensus that was described in the slogan, "Give Once for All." Laidlaw's reach spanned all levels of the community. For example, he drew avid support from both automotive titan Henry Ford II and pioneering labor leader Walter Reuther. In 1968, Laidlaw retired from his influential role in the organization, and by the 1970s, the phrase "United Way" was becoming widely adopted by the semi-independent affiliates in this worldwide network.

In the late 1980s, criticism arose concerning the way funds were being used in a number of the huge network's American affiliates. At the same time, United Way was facing declines in the automatic donations that had been provided by employees of large corporations since after World War II. As SIF publications describe United Way's history, the organization's 2007 commitment to a new "Community Impact Agenda" was a game-changer in the wake of these problems that had surfaced. One SIF report describes that 2007 change in focus as, "a vision for how United Ways could rebuild trust and remain credible, relevant, and effective." The SIF's analysis continues: "In this vision, United Way affiliates would target a limited number of issues and basic needs whose existence or lack thereof causes or contributes to poverty in communities across the country: income, education, and health. They would look beyond themselves and their network to partner with other grant makers, government agencies, corporations, and nonprofits to concentrate and magnify collective action and investment to tackle difficult social problems."

That's why SIF reports indicate that United Way organizations have proven to be effective partners in this kind of innovative, collaborative program. One SIF report describes the new United Way thinking this way: "United Way would no longer simply write checks to charities and hope they would do what they said they would do; rather, United Way would engage with recipients to strengthen their capacity to implement strong programs. These relationships would move beyond transactional to be transformational." As a result, since 2010, the SIF has funded work through United Way affiliates in parts of Louisiana, Minnesota, Colorado, Ohio, South Carolina, Oregon and Michigan.

However, as anyone who has worked in the nonprofit sector knows, not all grants are immediately accepted. United Way for Southeastern Michigan began its efforts to receive SIF funding in 2010, but had to retool its application before successfully applying in 2011. If you are considering applying for grants, remember that it takes time, sometimes a period measured in years, and you may need to make repeated attempts, even with a first-rate organization supporting your work.

Overall, the benefits of this partnership have been substantial. A SIF *Lessons and Stories* report describes the impact on the Metro Detroit organization this way:

> The SIF experience had transformative impacts on United Way for Southeastern Michigan (UWSEM) and its sub-grantees. It changed how UWSEM selects grantees, fostered a culture of data-informed decision-making, and bolstered formal and informal knowledge sharing.
>
> "SIF has had both direct and indirect impacts on the way that education work is being done here," said

Jennifer Callans, UWSEM's early education director. "The difference between our work before SIF and after is like night and day." ...

UWSEM needed to adapt to the SIF's rigorous evaluation requirements by building capacity for itself and for its sub-grantees in key areas such as data management. UWSEM also needed to align the evaluation activities of its sub-grantees, each of which had its own evaluation plan, third-party evaluator, and data system. To aggregate these different efforts, it worked with its sub-grantees and its portfolio evaluator, Child Trends, to create a common set of outcomes and indicators to serve as the basis for tracking progress across all programs.

If you are reading this book in hopes of launching or expanding a program in your community, many connected with the SIF advise that you first take a close look at the way you collect data about your program and then use it to evaluate your work in an ongoing way. Again, from the Metro Detroit section of the *Lessons and Stories* report:

The experience with data collection for the SIF grant was informative for everyone, including the sub-grantees, notes Jeffrey Miles, UWSEM's SIF manager.

> **Tip for Success: Climb Out of Your Silo**
> Big organizations like United Way can easily fall into silos. We might be funding an agency for something in education, something in basic needs and something in financial stability. Then, we realize all those United Way program officers need to be talking to each other. We've started convening cross-functional teams to share experiences with particular grantees across the organization.
> *From Jennifer Callans, UWSEM's early education director, in a SIF report.*

Tips from our portfolio evaluator

Child Trends, founded in 1979 and based in Bethesda, Maryland, is a leading nonprofit research organization focused on improving public policies and interventions that serve children and families. Programs funded by the SIF are required to conduct rigorous evaluation of their effectiveness, and one part of that effort at UWSEM was to contract with Child Trends, which would conduct ongoing interviews and analysis. The following tips are paraphrased from an interim report by Child Trends, drawing on extensive interviews with professionals working in the various SIF programs in the Detroit area. Although specifically focused on these programs in Southeast Michigan, these tips may be useful to anyone developing such programs in the future.

- **Clear and timely communication is essential.** Good communication is one key to success. Because UWSEM administers various SIF programs, the individual groups developing these programs depend on UWSEM for clear directions and compliance information, as well as updates. Communication also is important in the other direction – so that individual programs can voice their concerns, questions and challenges. One key step UWSEM took was to mandate a series of regular meetings to share updates and to hear what the participants were learning across the spectrum of these local programs.
- **Balance rigor with feasibility when it comes to evaluation plans for the new programs.** All SIF grants require evaluation plans, because the SIF's practice is to support and, ideally, to replicate programs that have clear evidence of success. At the same time, organizers need to understand how these evaluation activities may shape program implementation, which in turn may affect findings in the evaluation. This is a challenging aspect of participating in such a grant, and the six Detroit-area

programs all found that they had to pay a great deal of attention to meeting this goal. Organizations trying to develop such programs should not try to go it alone. They should meet as a team, discuss, research and develop strategies that can lead to best practices in evaluating the programs – while, at the same time, not compromising program implementation.

- **Build or improve capacity for data collection and management.** Nonprofits participating in a program like this vary in their capacity to track and manage data. Some have an established data collection infrastructure; others merely collect demographic and/or attendance data. The wide range of capacity in data management poses a challenge to systematically collecting high-quality data across all of the participating programs. To improve data quality, organizations considering such programs should take a close look at their own data management systems and share ideas for improving the management of data with other participating nonprofits. Again, don't go it alone in trying to determine how you will manage your data, share best practices with other organizations to improve everyone's capacity.

- **Tailor expectations of scaling to each program's stage of development.** Everyone hopes that good ideas will flourish and that effective programs will expand, but scaling depends on a program's stage of development. Whether programs ultimately prove effective or not, the fact is that programs don't all develop at the same rate. Some have greater barriers to overcome, while many programs must iron out a long series of glitches. Programs that are relatively new to an organization or community may need to gain experience before they can take off and have a smooth ride. It's critically important to realize that not all programs, even effective ones, will scale at the same rate.

- **Address ongoing funding challenges through collective problem solving.** Detroit is an example of an urban area with limited resources for funding and many nonprofits competing for dollars. UWSEM recognizes that challenge and helps to facilitate funding opportunities. But, even with the best intentions, such efforts sometimes do not prove fruitful. Raising local funds is one of the toughest challenges in this kind of work. Organizations considering such programs should try to find out how other similar communities are tackling this widespread problem. Sharing advice and opportunities on fundraising leverages collective problem-solving to address this major issue. By collaborating and sharing ideas with other community leaders, you may discover approaches that will help the entire community.

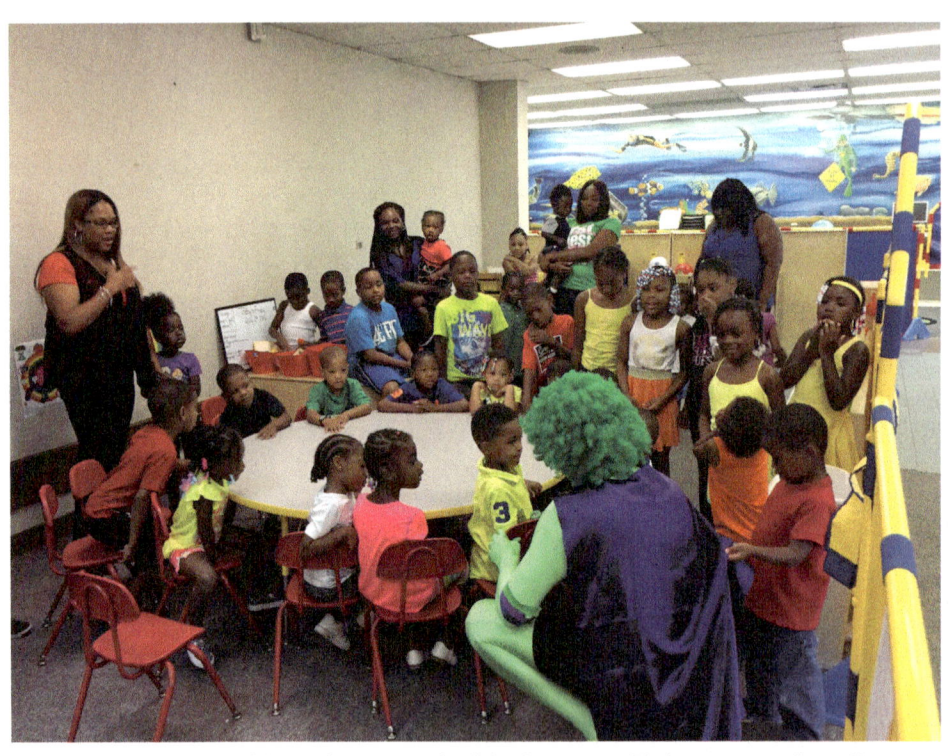

Regie talks with children about his colorful adventures. To learn more about Regie and the National Kidney Foundation of Michigan, visit: http://nkfm.org/

Acknowledgements

The National Kidney Foundation of Michigan would like to thank the following organizations:

For their generous financial support, without which we would not be able to reach all of the children and families that we do: United Way for Southeastern Michigan, the Michigan Nutrition Network at the Michigan Fitness Foundation, the Michigan Department of Health and Human Services, the Colina Foundation, the Corporation for National Community Service as part of the Social Innovation Fund, the MGM Resorts Foundation, the Staples Foundation, the General Motors Foundation, the UnitedHealthcare Community Plan, the Karen Colina Wilson Foundation, The Kresge Foundation Employee Matching Gifts program and Champions for Healthy Kids.

We would also like to thank the following individuals and organizations for their thoughtful contributions to Regie's Rainbow Adventure®: Dr. Art Franke, Kris and Thomas Ferriter, John Barker, Becky Dorner and Associates, Whole Foods Market, Dr. Jerry Yee, Virginia Romano, Cynthia Shaw and Dr. Jerry and Emilie Dancik.

Finally, we are grateful for having the pleasure to work with David Crumm and Shaun Taft, without whose hard work and support this book would not have been possible. Thank you for highlighting Regie's Rainbow Adventure and for helping us find the perfect way to communicate our passion for our program to others.

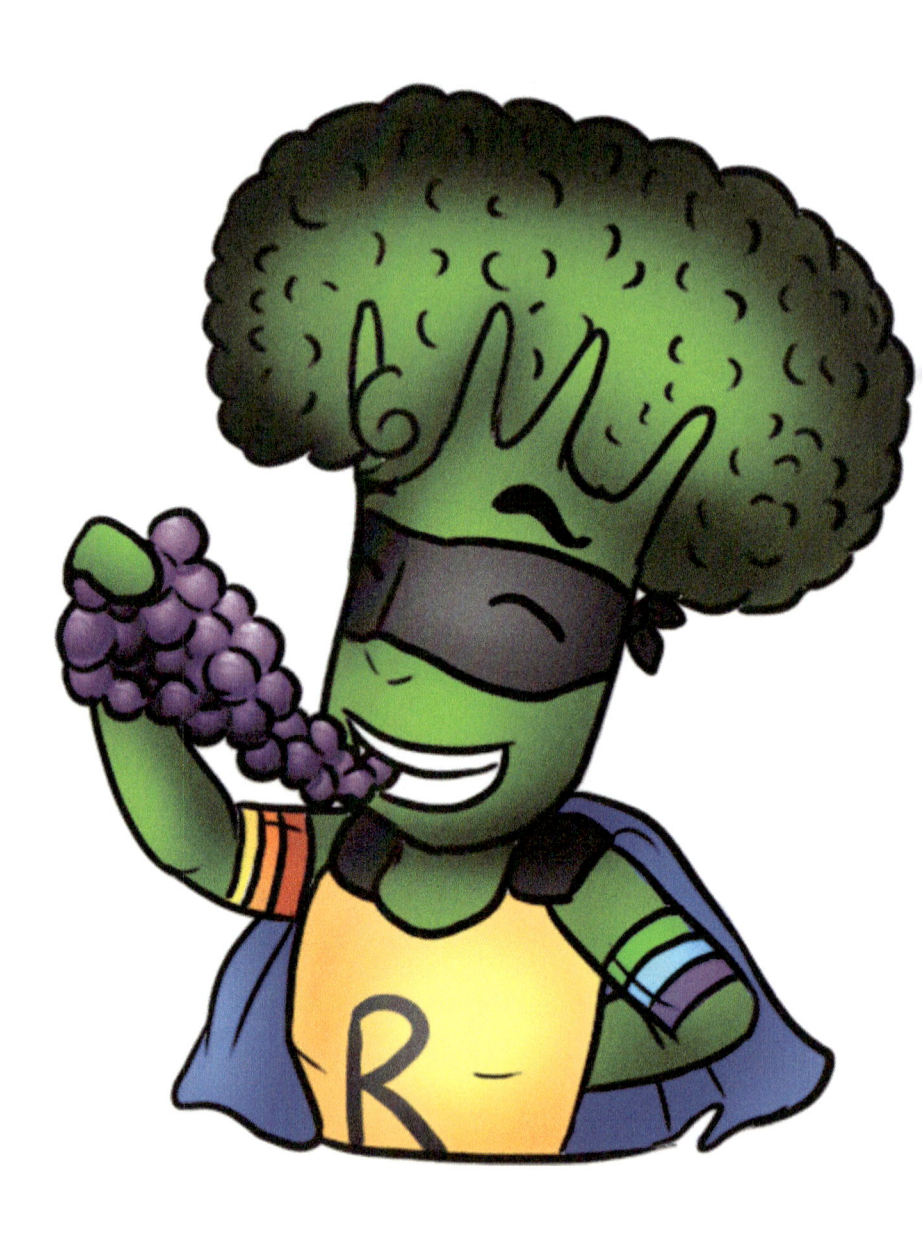

Regie on the Island of Purple.

About the Authors

Linda Smith-Wheelock currently serves as the executive vice president and chief operating officer at the National Kidney Foundation of Michigan (NKFM). She will become the president and chief executive officer in 2017. Linda is a licensed social worker and earned her Master of Social Work (M.S.W.) from the University of Michigan. She also earned her Master of Science (M.S.) in business administration from Madonna University. Linda oversees all programs including prevention programs, services to people with kidney disease, public health research and grant writing. Her favorite vegetable is green beans.

Crystal D'Agostino serves as program manager at the NKFM and is responsible for the oversight of all early childhood programming there, including the Regie's Rainbow Adventure program. Crystal began working for the NKFM in 2009, when her passion for kidney disease prevention and youth-based programming merged with Regie's Rainbow Adventure. Since then, she has successfully implemented and overseen this program in over 170 early childhood centers throughout the state. Crystal earned her Master of Social Work (M.S.W.) from Western Michigan University. Her favorite fruit is watermelon!

Maria Houroian serves as a program coordinator for the early childhood programs at the NKFM and is the program lead for Regie's Rainbow Adventure. She started her work with the NKFM as an intern and was so passionate about nutrition and improving the health of children that she became a full-time staff member three years ago. One of her favorite things, as a staff member, has been working with other team members in developing and updating Regie materials. Maria earned her Master of Social Work (M.S.W.) from Wayne State University with a concentration in community organizing. Her favorite vegetable is avocado!

Monica Easterling is a registered dietitian nutritionist and earned her master's degree in science. Monica has worked in various areas of the nutrition field and has served as nutrition manager for the New St. Paul Tabernacle Head Start Agency,

Inc. for the past 19 years. Monica has been a champion in promoting Regie's Rainbow Adventure within her Head Start sites, making sure that the program is implemented in a timely and efficient manner. She works with the centers' cooks, teachers and other staff to reinforce the Regie message of increasing fruit and vegetable intake and being more physically active. Her favorite fruit is pineapple.

The Bib to Backpack Learning Series

Join us in giving children a great start! Remember: Education begins before school. Research shows that the years between the bib and the backpack make all the difference for school readiness and lifelong success. So, let's make those years count!

That's our goal at United Way for Southeastern Michigan in launching this new campaign we call Bib to Backpack. A wide range of informational resources are available for parents and caregivers online at: www.BibToBackpack.org.

In addition, this Learning Series within the campaign will expand into six individual books throughout 2016, highlighting the inspiring and innovative programs we are sponsoring through the Corporation for National and Community Service's Social Innovation Fund. Sharing these programs with other communities is a major goal of that fund's important work nationwide. We hope that the stories, voices and resources in these books will inspire parents, students, community leaders and professionals nationwide who are looking for fresh ideas to prepare children for school.

Related Books

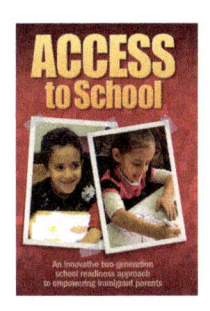

ACCESS to School:
An innovative two-generation school readiness approach to empowering immigrant parents
In this book, you will read about immigrant parents seeking a better life for their children with help from American educators. ACCESS and the other learning communities hope readers will learn from their accomplishments, then will use some of these ideas to shape their own programs.
www.BibToBackpack.org
ISBN: 978-1-942011-26-2

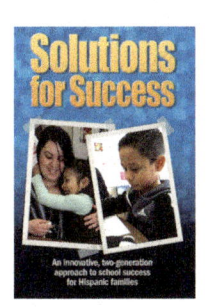

Solutions for Success:
An innovative, two generation approach to school success for Hispanic families
We are a nation of immigrants. In this book, you'll discover an innovative program in Detroit that teaches Hispanic-immigrant parents English while these parents also are ensuring their children's success at school.
www.BibToBackpack.org
ISBN: 978-1-942011-46-0

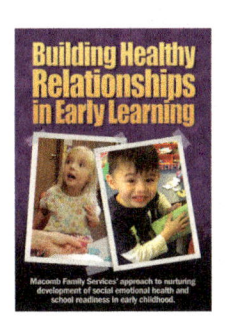

Building Healthy Relationships in Early Learning:
Macomb Family Services' approach to nurturing development of social emotional healthy and school readiness in early childhood.
Join Macomb Family Services as you learn about the journey that has cultivated a multi-disciplinary network of relationships supporting children's social-emotional health and school readiness.
www.BibToBackpack.org
ISBN: 978-1-942011-57-6

Print and ebooks available from Amazon.com and other retailers.

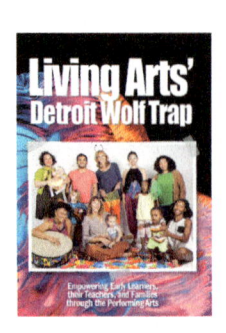

Living Arts' Detroit Wolf Trap:
Empowering Early Learners, their Teachers, and Families through the Performing Arts.
This is the inspiring story of artists, trained in early childhood education. It's the story of the Detroit non-profit Living Arts, which now is a national affiliate of the Wolf Trap Institute for Early Learning through the Arts.
www.BibToBackpack.org
ISBN: 978-1-942011-61-3

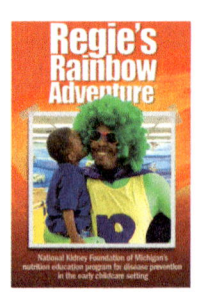

Regie's Rainbow Adventure:
National Kidney Foundation of Michigan's nutrition education program for disease prevention in the early childcare setting
Regie's Rainbow Adventure® tells the amazing story of a team of creative professionals who created a broccoli-shaped superhero to carry their message of healthy eating and physical activity to preschool-aged children.
www.BibToBackpack.org
ISBN: 978-1-942011-64-4

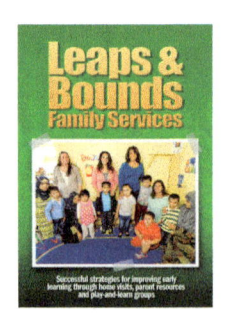

Leaps & Bounds Family Services:
Successful strategies for improving early learning through home visits, parent resources and play-and-learn groups
"Small and mighty"—that's the reputation of Michigan-based Leaps & Bounds Family Services, an early-learning nonprofit that is highly respected as a successful example of sustainability, collaboration and effectiveness in responding to community needs.
www.BibToBackpack.org
ISBN: 978-1-942011-67-5

Print and ebooks available from Amazon.com and other retailers.